LAPAROSCOPY
FOR
SURGEONS

LAPAROSCOPY FOR SURGEONS

Barry A. Salky, M.D., F.A.C.S.

Clinical Associate Professor of Surgery
Mount Sinai School of Medicine
New York, New York

With Contribution by

George Berci, M.D., F.A.C.S.

Associate Director of Surgery
Cedars-Sinai Medical Center
And
Clinical Professor of Surgery
UCLA School of Medicine
Los Angeles, California

IGAKU-SHOIN New York • Tokyo

Published and distributed by

IGAKU-SHOIN Medical Publishers, Inc.
1140 Avenue of the Americas, New York, N.Y. 10036

IGAKU-SHOIN Ltd.,
5-24-3 Hongo, Bunkyo-ku, Tokyo

Library of Congress Cataloging-in-Publication Data

Salky, Barry A.
Laparoscopy for surgeons / Barry A. Salky.
p. cm.
1. Abdomen—Surgery. 2. Laparoscopy. I. Title.
[DNLM: 1. Peritoneoscopy—atlases. WI 17 S186L]
RD540.S25 1990
617.5′507545—dc20
DNLM/DLC
for Library of Congress 90-4134
CIP

ISBN: 0-89640-166-9 (New York)
ISBN: 4-260-14166-X (Tokyo)

Printed and bound in the U.S.A.

10 9 8 7 6 5 4 3 2 1

To Alma, Jonathan, and Adam—
need I say more?

PREFACE

When I think back to 8 years ago while I was performing my first laparoscopy, I remember how close I came to forgetting this procedure completely. Three liters of nitrous oxide in the preperitoneal space produces significant subcutaneous crepitations. Fortunately, my next several laparoscopies demonstrated quite clearly to me the beauty of this procedure. It became obvious that laparoscopy is a technique ideally suited to abdominal surgeons because of their operative experience and their firsthand knowledge of gross pathology. The surgeon does not have to learn the difference between right and left lobes of the liver, where the falciform ligament is located, or the varied positions of the appendix, for example. It has been my experience that the major impediment to the use of the laparoscope by general surgeons is that surgeons do not really understand how the laparoscope can be used effectively. Most surgeons are not exposed to this technique during their training and would, therefore, not be expected to give it high priority. The gastrointestinal and surgical literature has very few references describing its usefulness to the general surgeon. In short, this highly accurate, low-morbidity technique has been neglected by the practitioners who would be able to use it best. It is my hope that this atlas, purposely slanted for the general surgeon, will allow surgeons to more fully appreciate laparoscopy's usefulness. I have set up the text to follow actual clinical cases in which I have been personally involved. The text describes the reasoning behind the decision for performing each laparoscopy. I hope that this atlas provides a starting point for my fellow surgeons and that its use increases as surgeons gain familiarity with it.

Therapeutic laparoscopy is rapidly breaking new ground. Recent advances in instrumentation (video, high-flow insufflators, automatic laparoscopic clip applicators, etc.) and inventiveness by some of our surgical colleagues have made laparoscopic cholecystectomy possible. Towards the end of chapter 6, I will describe one of the techniques for performing this innovative procedure. I truly believe it marks the beginning of a new frontier for laparoscopic surgery.

I would sincerely like to thank Drs. William Boyd and Worth Boyce for introducing the laparoscope and the techniques for using it to me. They are doctors who care deeply about doing the right thing and teaching it to others.

Barry A. Salky, M.D.

CONTENTS

1. INSTRUMENTATION AND TECHNIQUE **1**

2. ABDOMINAL PAIN **17**

3. ABDOMINAL MASSES **45**

4. LIVER DISEASE **59**

5. ASCITES **99**

6. THERAPEUTIC LAPAROSCOPY **113**

7. EMERGENCY LAPAROSCOPY **145**
George Berci

8. APPENDIX **153**

INDEX **155**

1

INSTRUMENTATION AND TECHNIQUE

The classical indications for performing laparoscopy are listed on page 2 in Table 1.1. As the reader can tell, the surgeon has firsthand knowledge from operative experience of nearly all of the indications shown. In the author's experience, this allows the surgeon a decided advantage in appreciating the visual findings at laparoscopy. This in turn will make for a high diagnostic capability for the surgeon performing the procedure. While some of the diagnoses are not truly surgical diseases, the invasiveness of the procedure and the anatomic relationships make the surgeon ideally suited to this modality. As with any newly acquired technique, a learning curve is to be expected. However, in the author's experience, this curve is not steep or long, given the basic surgical practices attained during a surgical residency program.

The contraindications are just as important as the indications, and they are listed in Table 1.2. The risk of perforation upon introduction of the Veress needle or laparoscopic trocar is high in intestinal obstruction. The potential development of incarceration by a displaced viscous makes this procedure dangerous in patients with an associated large diaphragmatic hernia. Abdominal wall hernias do not present a problem. The development of fascitis is possible in patients with abdominal

Table 1-1 INDICATIONS

Abdominal pain, acute and chronic
Focal liver disease
Abdominal masses
Abdominal trauma
Ascites of unknown etiology
Therapeutic

wall infections. Therefore, the infection should be controlled before undertaking laparoscopy. Coagulation defects of a mild degree (protime no more than 4 sec) are usually not a problem if no biopsy is planned. However, if a biopsy is needed, strict normalization of any coagulopathy must be accomplished beforehand. Previous surgery is only a relative contraindication. In the author's experience, 40% of patients have had at least one previous surgical procedure, and several patients have had multiple operations. In general, uncooperative patients and young patients should be laparoscoped under general anesthesia, as good cooperation is needed during the performance of laparoscopy to ensure its safety.

Table 1-2 CONTRAINDICATIONS

Absolute	*Relative*
Intestinal obstruction	Mild coagulapathy
Abdominal wall infection	Uncooperative patient
Uncorrectable coagulapathy	Diaphragmatic hernia

INSTRUMENTATION

There have been significant advances in the optics and illumination capacities that now allow an excellent visualization of the abdominal cavity through a rigid laparoscope. A variety of different sized laparoscopes, ranging from 3 mm to 10 mm in diameter, is also available, depending on the needs of the surgeon. There are several companies that supply these instruments, and the choice should be based on the surgeon's preference. In general, the major components (laparoscope and light source) are not interchangeable. The following instrumentation has worked well for the author in terms of its simplicity, reliability, and photographic documentation.

The spring-loaded Veress insufflation needle (Fig. 1.1) is designed to minimize inadvertant injury to the underlying bowel. The standard 100-mm length needle is used routinely, although a 120-mm needle is available for obese patients. There are various-sized trocars and sleeves for

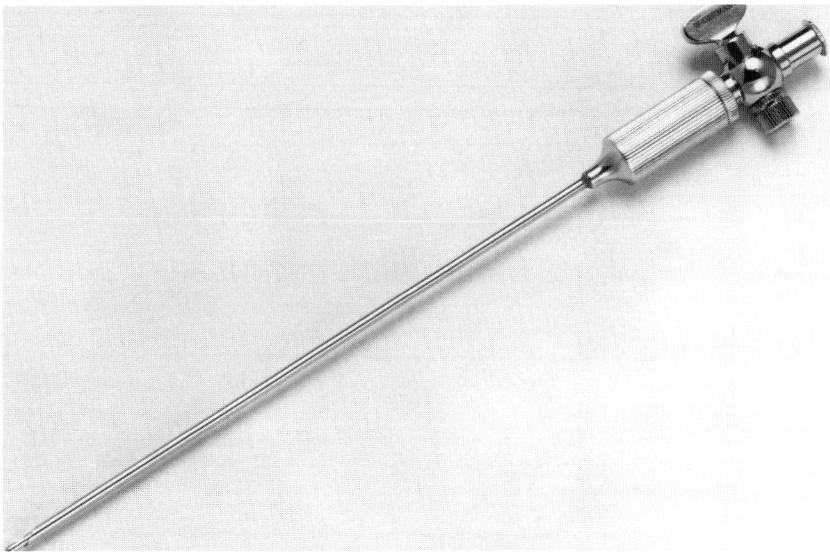

Figure 1.1
Veress pneumoperitoneum needle is shown assembled with stop-cock gas valve and Leur lock female attachment.

puncture of the abdominal wall, each appropriate for a standard telescope. The author prefers the 10-mm size in the routine patient (nonoperated), as the photographic capabilities are better with the larger telescopes. Figure 1.2 demonstrates the two trocar tips available. The author prefers the pyramidal style because of its ease of insertion. Whichever tip is used, it should be sharp. As stated earlier, the 10-mm telescope is used routinely, unless multiple previous surgeries have been performed, increasing the likelihood of extensive adhesions. The author will then use the 5-mm-long telescope to further decrease the chance of injury (Fig. 1.3). A variety of ancillary instruments is also available for use through the second puncture site (Fig. 1.4). They are supplied for either 3-mm or 5-mm sleeves. A palpating probe, lancet-shaped biopsy forceps, 18-gauge aspirating needle, and bipolar locking-grasping forceps are also needed to complete the basic instrumentation set (Fig. 1.5).

Illumination is provided by the Olympus CLE-F light source (Fig. 1.6). Figure 1.7 demonstrates the fiber optic cable attached to the 10-mm telescope. The male end of the cable is inserted into the female receptacle on the light source. The halogen bulb inside the light source provides exceptional brightness, which is transmitted through the cable to the telescope. Near perfect photographic documentation is possible with the Olympus OM-2 SLR camera outfitted with the OM-12 endoscopic screen and SM-EFR lens adapter. Kodak Ektachrome ASA 400-slide film is used routinely (Fig. 1.8). The system is completely automated so that the

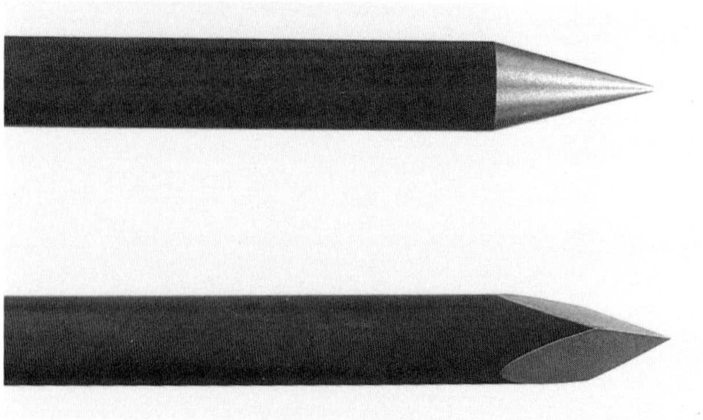

Figure 1.2
Top: Conical shaped trocar tip; Bottom: Pyramidal shaped trocar tip.

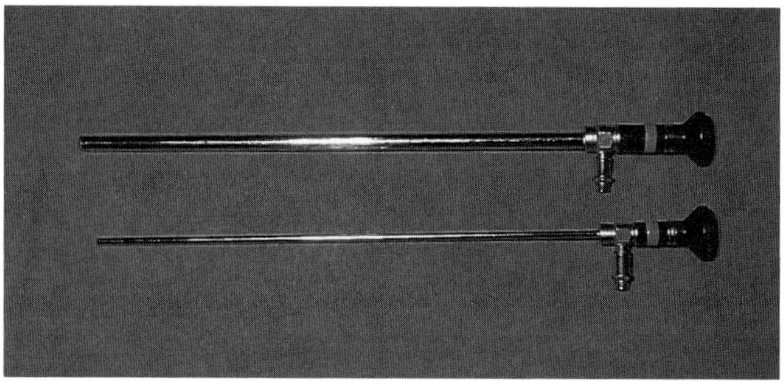

Figure 1.3
Top: 10 mm 0° angle telescope; Bottom: 5 mm 5° angle telescope.

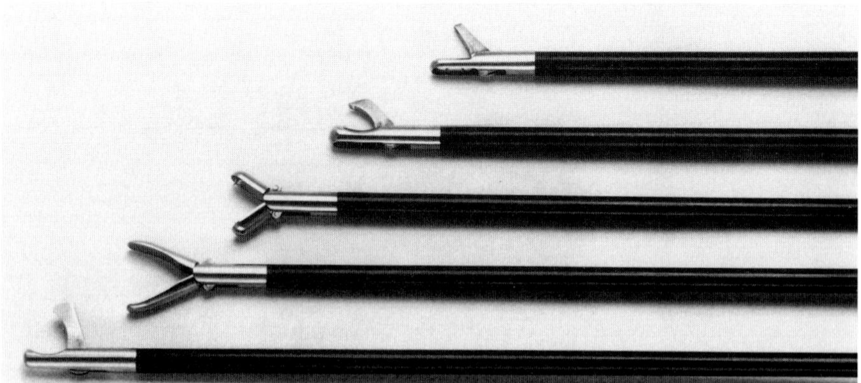

Figure 1.4
From top to bottom, the first three instruments are punch biopsy forceps with cutting jaws. The fourth instrument is a tissue forceps used for grasping and specimen retrieval. The last instrument is a hook-scissor used for adhesion lysis.

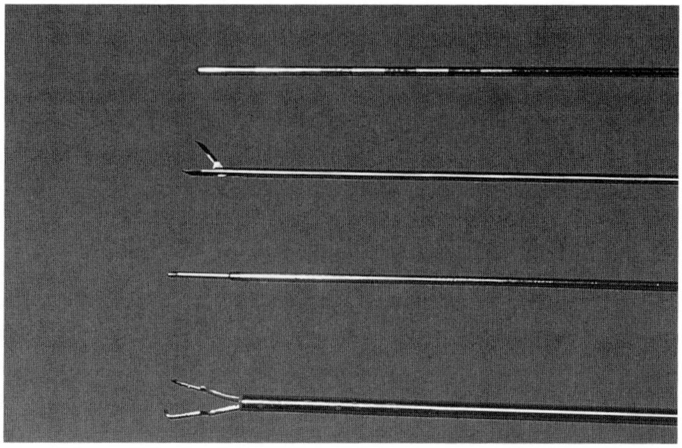

Figure 1.5
From top to bottom, a 3 mm palpating probe marked in 1 cm increments, a 5 mm palpating probe, a Lancet-shaped biopsy forceps, a 14-gauge, 3-mm-diameter aspirating needle, a Bipolar grasping forceps.

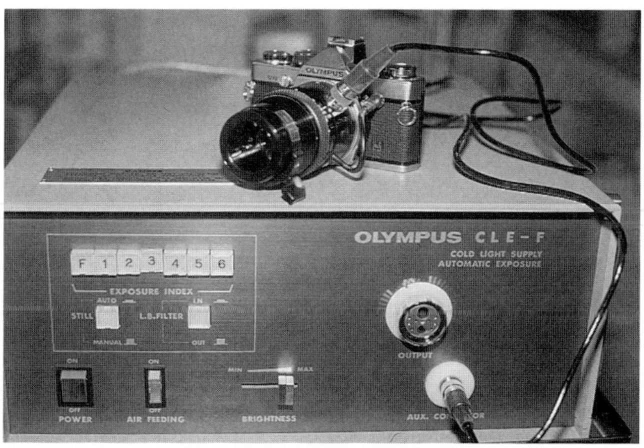

Figure 1.6
Olympus CLE-F light source. The Olympus OM-1 camera with cable connector attaches to the auxillary port. Exposure index is set to 3.

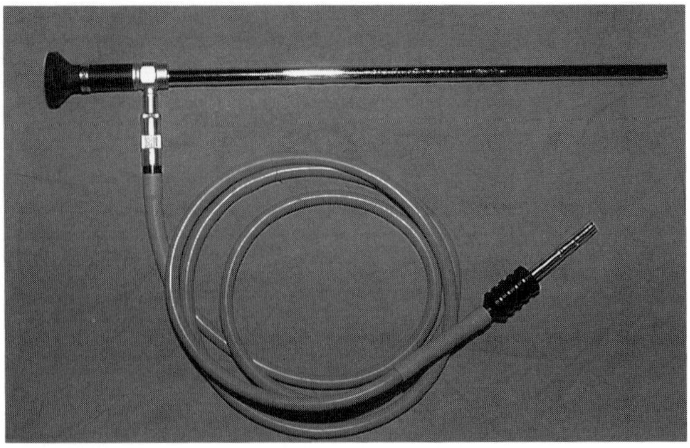

Figure 1.7
Olympus 10 mm rigid laparoscope with fiberoptic cable attached.

surgeon only has to focus and shoot. All color plates in this atlas were obtained with this system. Present technology now allows video (television) laparoscopy as well. This will permit more complex procedures in the years to come. (See Chapter 6, laparoscopic cholecystectomy.)

There are multiple insufflators on the market. The author has found them all to be about the same in terms of their safety and reliability.

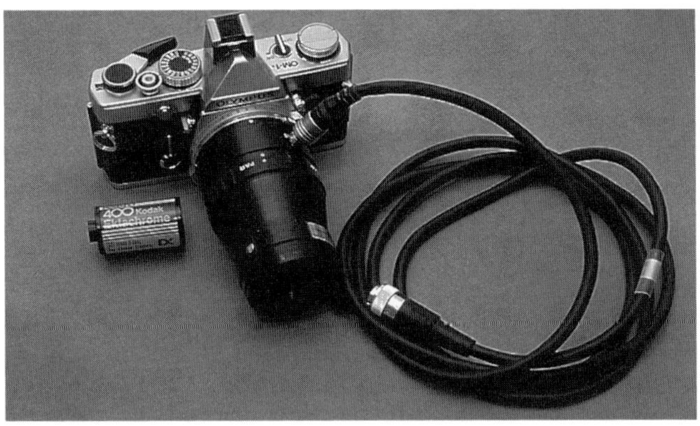

Figure 1.8
An Olympus OM-1 camera with SM-EFR and direct cable for attachment to light source. Ektachrome 400 ASA film is used routinely.

TECHNIQUE

Laparoscopy is usually performed in an endoscopy suite or operating room. A standard tilt endoscopic table or regular operating room table

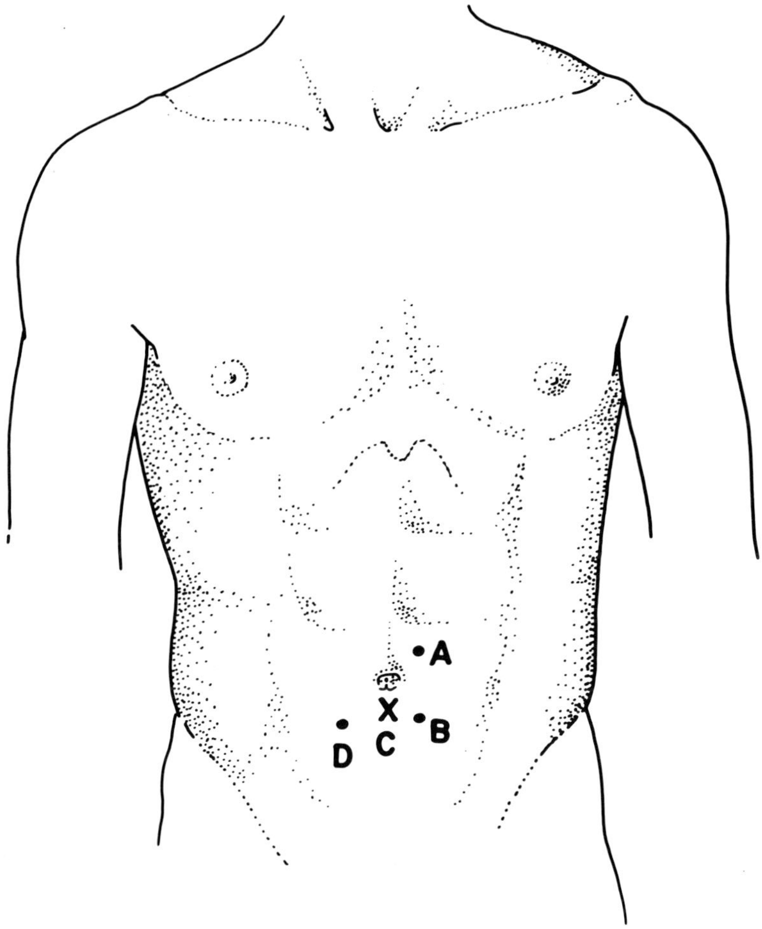

Figure 1.9
The author's preference is site A, however, sites A,B,C and D are safe for puncture.

will be sufficient. The patient is placed supine, and a povoiodine prep of the abdominal wall is done by means of standard sterile technique. Blood pressure and electrocardiogram are monitored by the nursing/ anesthesia staff while the procedure is taking place. This procedure can be performed at bedside in an emergency, but there is some limitation in hospital bed movement, which may impact on proper positioning of the patient.

Figure 1.9 illustrates the usual sites for insertion of the pneumoperitoneum needle (Veress). The author's preference is above and to the left of the umbilicus, if the procedure is being performed under local anesthesia. The right upper quadrant in the area of the round ligament usually has a significant amount of properitoneal fat, which makes penetration of the abdominal wall difficult, and should be avoided as an insertion site. The epigastric vessels are about 3 cm lateral to the midline and should be avoided as well. If the patient is under general anesthesia and there is no reason to expect the presence of collateral venous channels, the umbilical approach is used. If the patient has had previous surgery, the puncture site must be at least 1 cm away from the surgical scar. Therefore, depending on where the pathology is located, considerable variation of the "usual" puncture sites may be necessary.

Local anesthesia is preferable to general anesthesia for obvious reasons and is used routinely by the author in more than 90% of patients. However, if the patient is uncooperative or young, or a therapeutic undertaking that is painful to the patient is going to be used, general anesthesia should be used. On the average, 20 to 25 cc of 0.5% lidocaine are needed to produce complete anesthesia of the abdominal wall for painless insertion of the Veress needle. Figure 1.10 demonstrates the proper placement of local anesthesia in the abdominal wall. It is helpful to think in terms of a cone with the apex at the skin and the base at the parietal peritoneum. The relatively large base is necessary because the laparoscope will be rotated about the axis of the abdominal wall. This maneuver is painful unless adequate anesthesia is present. A 1-cm incision is made at the site of local anesthetic placement. The subcutaneous fat is bluntly separated down to the anterior rectus fascia by using a hemostat. The patient is asked to tense and push out the abdominal wall. The Veress pneumoperitoneum needle is inserted at right angles to the fascia. Two distinct "pops" can be heard as the anterior rectus fascia and posterior fascia–parietal peritoneum layers are penetrated. A small amount of saline (5 cc) is injected into the Veress needle, and the syringe is removed. If the Veress needle is in proper position, the meniscus of saline should be pulled into the peritoneal cavity with a deep inspiration and, therefore, will no longer be visible at the hub of the Veress needle. If the meniscus is still present, the Veress needle is not in good position, and the insufflation of gas should not begin. Either choose another site or replace the needle. This occurrence is not that uncommon in a previously operated abdomen, and it is one of the main reasons why 0.5% lidocaine is used. If another site is needed, toxic levels of local anesthesia will not be a problem.

Once the proper position of the Veress needle is confirmed, insufflation is started. Nitrous oxide is the insufflation gas of choice. The normally present small amount of peritoneal fluid does not react to the nitrous oxide. Therefore, there is no peritoneal irritation from the gas. Carbon dioxide, which is the more common gas used for gynecological laparoscopy, will combine with the peritoneal fluid to form weak carbonic acid that is irritating to the parietal peritoneum. As most of the

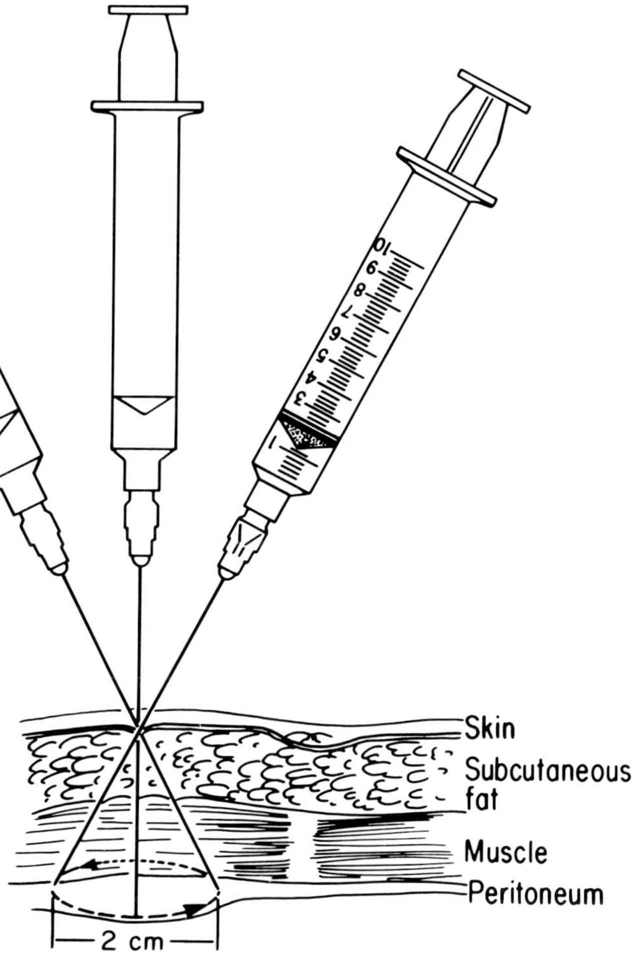

Figure 1.10
Local anesthesia is placed in a cone-shaped fashion with the base at the peritoneum.

patients are awake, this can cause significant patient discomfort. The amount of nitrous gas absorbed by the peritoneum is negligible.

The Veress needle is attached to the insufflator via standard suction tubing. The intraabdominal pressure is continuously monitored. Ideally, the pressure should be less than 20 mm Hg. In thin patients, it is usually 10 to 12 mm Hg. Obesity or tense ascites will elevate the pressure. If the pressure is not satisfactory, the surgeon must stop the insufflation and ascertain the cause of the high pressure. The common reasons are omentum or bowel partially occluding the Veress needle, the Veress needle has been placed too deep and is abutting the posterior peritoneum, or the Veress needle is still in the abdominal wall. All of the above just require repositioning of the needle. If the reason for the high pressure can not be explained, the procedure should be abandoned. The initial insufflation should be on manual (see insufflator toggle switches). As soon as the desired amount of gas is placed in the free peritoneal space (usually at least 2000 cc), the switch is changed to automatic. This will allow the pneumoperitoneum to stay at the desired level while the various instruments are placed in and out of the abdomen. There is a flow valve that will allow a visual check of the gas as it is insufflated into the patient. It is the same as a standard anesthesia machine. A special note about ascitic patients is necessary. If the gas is blown into the ascites, large "soap-like" bubbles will form that will preclude proper visualization. This can be obviated by placing the Veress needle parallel to the abdominal wall (Fig. 1.11) and insufflating approximately 300 to 500 cc of gas to form a small cupula. The needle can then be rotated to a more perpendicular position without fear of causing bubbles.

The Veress needle is removed, and the laparoscopic trocar and sleeve are positioned perpendicular to the rectus fascia for insertion. The sleeve and trocar are grasped firmly in the palm of the dominate hand. The fingers of the other hand should be positioned about three-quarters of the distance from the end of the sleeve to prevent an inadvertent deep penetration of the abdominal wall by the trocar (Fig. 1.12). The trocar tip should be sharp, which significantly facilitates its passage through the abdominal wall. The patient then simultaneously tenses and pushes out the abdominal wall. The trocar and sleeve are then pushed into the free peritoneal space. A distinct "pop" will be felt as the instrument penetrates the posterior fascia. The pressure required to penetrate the abdominal wall should be delivered as a quick burst rather than slow and steady. If the latter is used, there is a much higher incidence of intra-

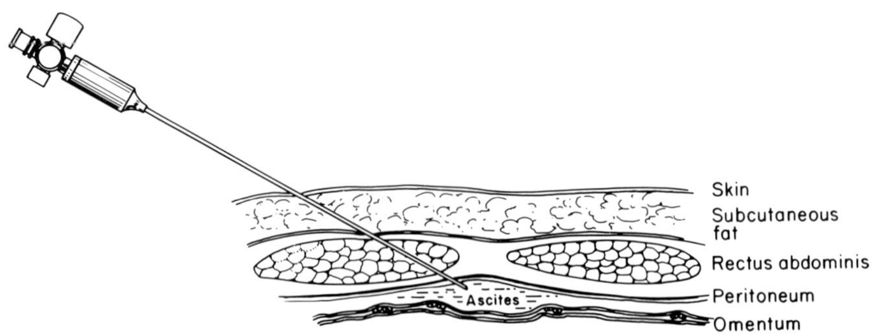

Figure 1.11
The relatively parallel position of the Veress needle to the abdominal wall is shown.

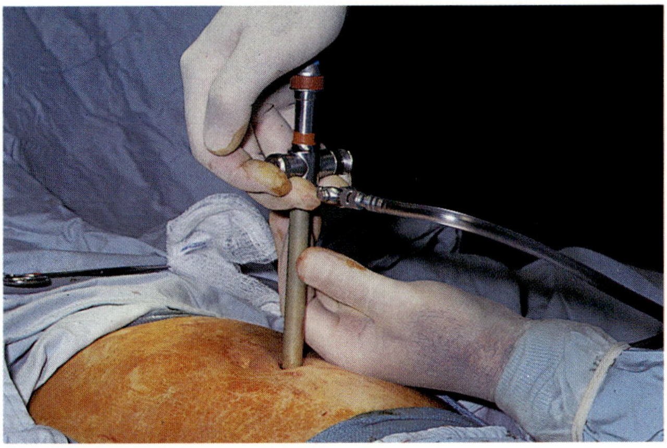

Figure 1.12
The back of the surgeon's left hand is resting on the abdominal wall. When the patient tenses the abdominal muscles, the pressure is transmitted to the surgeon's hand. The sleeve is grasped three-quarters of the way up between the thumb and the index finger. The sleeve and trocar are held firmly in the palm of the surgeon's right hand.

abdominal injury as the abdominal wall is compressed between the trocar and the spine. It is important to instruct the patient before the procedure in the mechanics of tensing and pushing out the abdominal wall at the same time. It is difficult for some patients to grasp. It also allays anxiety that patients often have about the procedure.

Once the surgeon has inserted the trocar and sleeve into the peritoneal space, the trocar is removed. The suction tubing that was attached to the Veress needle and the insufflator is now connected to the laparoscopic sleeve. The intraabdominal pressure will now be readable on the insufflator. The pressure should fluctuate with respiration and be 20 mm Hg or less. If there are no respiratory fluctuations, the sleeve is not in the abdominal cavity. This will be confirmed when the laparoscope is inserted through the sleeve. The trocar will need to be reinserted and more pressure applied to enter the peritoneal space. High pressure should alert the surgeon to the same problem, or there has been an injury to the bowel, and the sleeve is in the intestines. Direct inspection of the underlying structures beneath the puncture site is performed first. Any trauma to the omentum or bowel must be identified before proceeding to performance of the laparoscopy. Once an atraumatic insertion has been confirmed visually, the laparoscope is directed toward the falciform ligament in order to properly orient the surgeon (Fig. 1.13). A second puncture trocar and sleeve are then inserted into the peritoneal cavity under direct vision after placement of local anesthesia. Figures

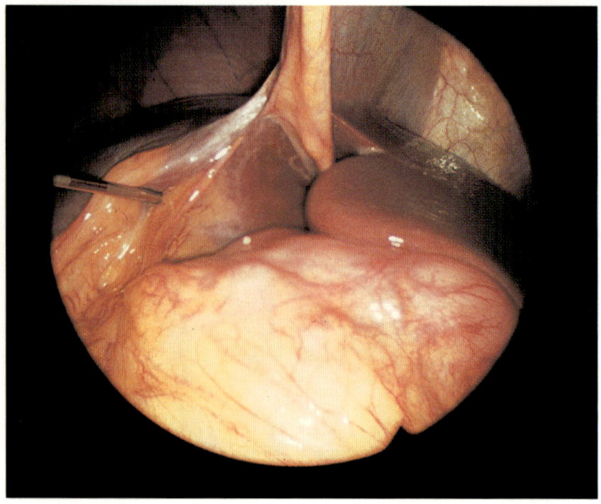

Figure 1.13
The ligamentum teres and falciform ligament separating the medial and lateral segments of the left lobe are clearly seen at the top of the figure. The central tendon of the diaphragm is in the background, and the stomach is in the foreground. A second puncture probe is visible on the left.

1.14**A** and **B** demonstrate the appropriate wheal produced by the administration of the local. The site of the puncture is variable, depending on where the pathology is located. The trocar is removed, and a palpating probe is inserted. A thorough examination of the abdominal cavity is not possible without a palpating probe, and, in the author's opinion, it is mandatory. The surgeon then proceeds in an orderly sequence around the peritoneal cavity for a general inspection. Normal views of the left upper quadrant, left lower quadrant, pelvis, right lower quadrant, and right upper quadrant as seen in Figs. 1.15–1.19, respectively. It is common to find unsuspected pathology that may impact on the patient's prognosis. Therefore, inspection of as much of the abdominal cavity as possible is always performed. The undersurface of the left lobe of the liver can not be seen without lifting it up with a palpating probe (Fig. 1.20). In this case, a benign cyst is evident. It is a commonplace to harbor metastatic disease which, when found, may preclude formal liver resection.

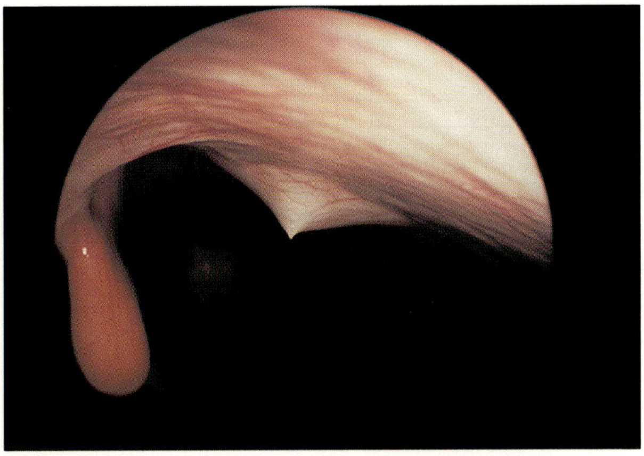

Figure 1.14A
View of the left upper quadrant demonstrating local anesthetic wheal placement. The tip of the needle is almost visible. The round ligament is seen to the left.

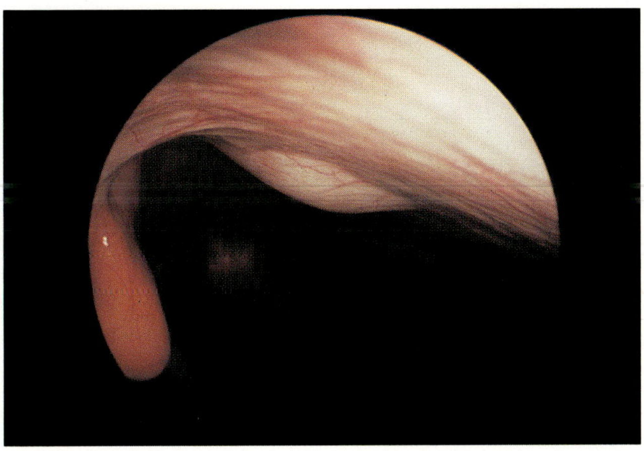

Figure 1.14B
Two centimeter wheal in the parietal peritoneum seen.

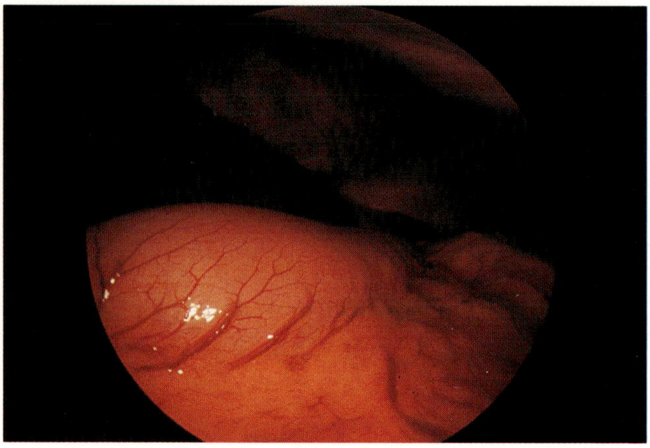

Figure 1.15
Left upper quadrant view demonstrating lateral segment of left lobe resting on the stomach. The greater curvature of the stomach with its gastroepiploic blood vessels are clearly seen. The greater omentum is also demonstrated. The left hemidiaphragm is in the background.

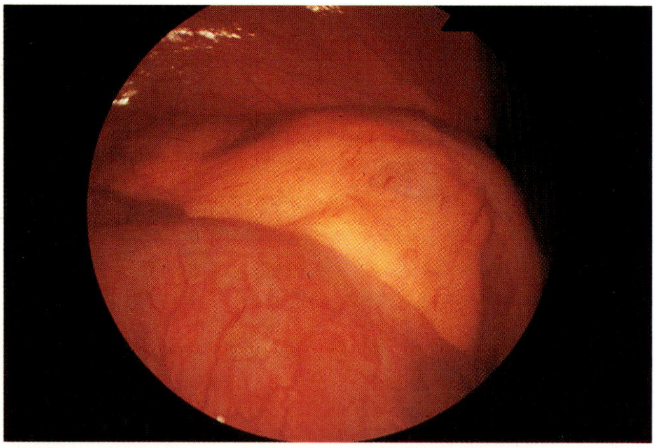

Figure 1.16
View of the left lower quadrant demonstrating a loop of small intestine in the foreground and the sigmoid colon in the background. A tenia coli is clearly seen on the sigmoid.

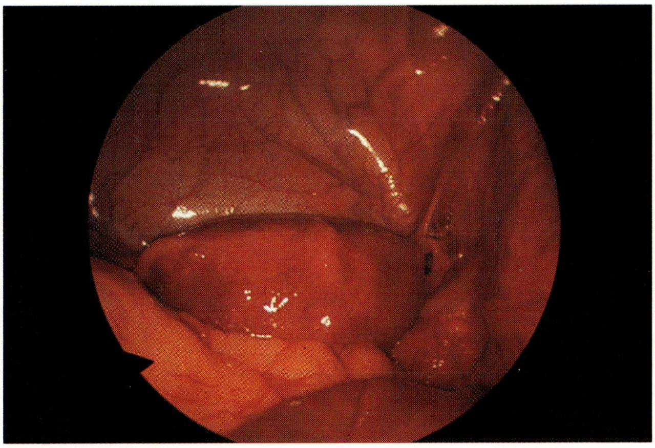

Figure 1.17
Pelvic view showing uterus with right adenexa visible. A loop of small intestine is just seen at the bottom, and the sigmoid colon is to the left. The parietal peritoneum covering an empty urinary bladder is visible above the uterus.

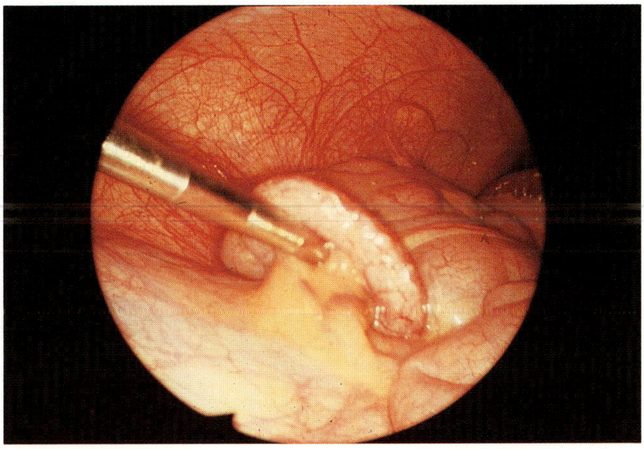

Figure 1.18
Right lower quadrant view showing appendix lifted up by a second puncture probe. The cecum and right parietal peritoneum is visible in the background, and a loop of small intestine is seen at the bottom right.

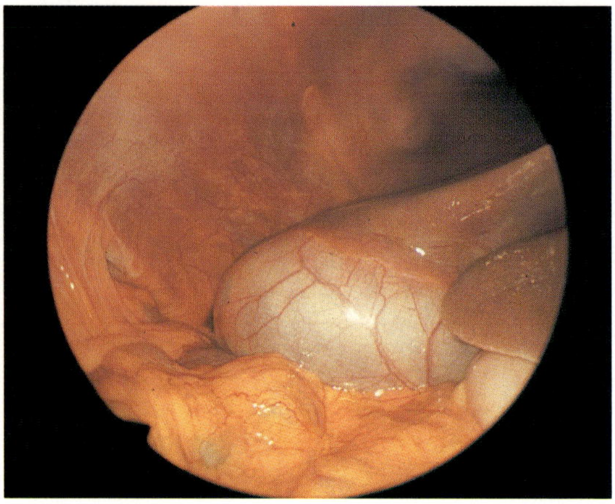

Figure 1.19
Right upper quadrant demonstrating a distended gall bladder and prominent cleft between the two let lobe segments. The hepatic flexure of the colon is seen in the foreground and the right hemidiaphragm is present in the background.

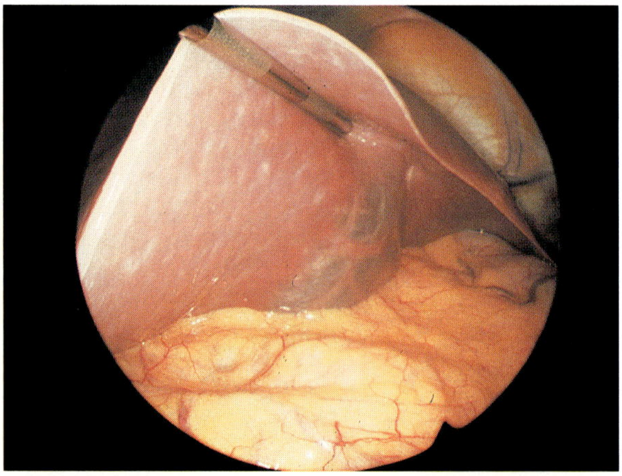

Figure 1.20
The under surface of the lateral segment of the left lobe is seen with upward displacement by the second puncture probe. The lesser omentum and part of the lesser curvature of the stomach is visible. A simple cyst of the liver is also seen. The left hemidiaphragm is in the background.

2

ABDOMINAL PAIN

The general surgeon is frequently called to evaluate patients with acute abdominal pain. In most instances, the etiology can be elucidated easily by integrating the patient's history, physical examination, laboratory data, and radiological studies. The surgeon's plan of action then proceeds accordingly. However, occasionally the correct diagnosis may not be clear based on the available information, and, therefore, the proper course to pursue may be in question. In some of these cases, the patients are extremely ill, or they have concurrent medical problems that would make an unneeded laparotomy risky. It is in these types of management problems that laparoscopy may be very useful. In this author's experience laparoscopy is 97% accurate in the diagnosis of acute abdominal pain syndromes. In most instances, laparoscopy is performed with local anesthesia, which carries a very low morbidity. In the intensive care unit setting, it may be performed at bedside.

Chronic abdominal pain is a frustrating problem for patient and surgeon alike. The patients frequently have had one or more previous surgeries. They have had multiple diagnostic evaluations by both noninvasive and invasive means without defining the problem. The economic drain on the patient is often considerable as well. In the author's experience, laparoscopy has defined the problem 55% of the time. In certain situations, therapeutic maneuvers through the laparoscope have been definitive. However, laparoscopy should be reserved for those patients in whom less invasive measures have failed to identify the problem. It is important to perform the procedure under local anesthesia, as the patient may be able to help with pain localization while the surgeon manipulates the viscera with the second puncture probe.

The following pictorial cases will describe in detail laparoscopy's usefulness to the surgeon.

ACUTE ABDOMINAL PAIN

The most frequent use of laparoscopy for acute abdominal pain is in the differential diagnosis of right lower quadrant pain. In the majority of cases, acute appendicitis is easily diagnosed based on all the usual parameters that surgeons follow. However, review of the surgical literature condones a "negative" appendectomy rate of approximately 10%, attesting to the occasional difficulty in making the proper diagnosis. Laparoscopy is an ideal procedure in just this setting.

Case 2.1

A 59-year-old female with fever and right lower quadrant (RLQ) pain. There was a known history of chronic myelogenous leukemia (CML). The WBC count was markedly elevated, consistent with CML. The palpating probe is seen lifting an inflamed appendix away from the cecum. The patient's low platelet count accounts for the hemorrhagic appearance. Dx: Acute appendicitis. Case 2.1 clearly demonstrates the advantage of laparoscopy in the differential diagnosis of acute RLQ pain. The

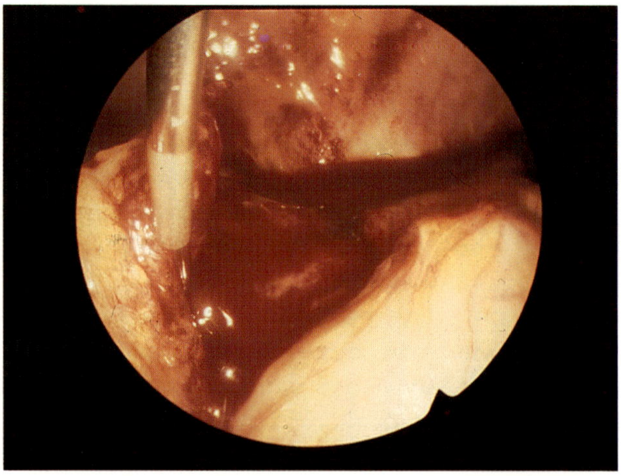

confirmation of a surgically correctable problem was gratifying in this patient's complicated medical situation. A negative laparotomy would likely have produced significant morbidity. The laparoscopy was performed under local anesthesia.

Case 2.2

A 32-year-old female with fever and RLQ peritoneal findings. She was on chemotherapy for Hodgkin's disease and was neutropenic. Pelvic examination revealed normal adnexa without cervical tenderness. A preoperative sonogram revealed fluid in the pelvis. Figure 2.2 reveals a pelvic hemoperitoneum. The second puncture palpating probe is lifting the right adnexa. The rectosigmoid colon is visible in the foreground. Although not seen in the picture, the appendix was entirely normal. There was a small amunt of blood in the RLQ. Dx: Ruptured ovarian cyst. Aspiration of the bloody fluid via the second puncture site relieved the pain. The procedure was performed under local anesthesia. Case 2.2 illustrates a nonsurgical cause of RLQ peritonitis in a very high-risk patient. Even though the clinical picture was one of "acute appendicitis," a negative laparotomy was prevented by the use of the laparoscope. Not only was the diagnosis established, but also therapeutic benefit was obtained by aspirating the irritating blood.

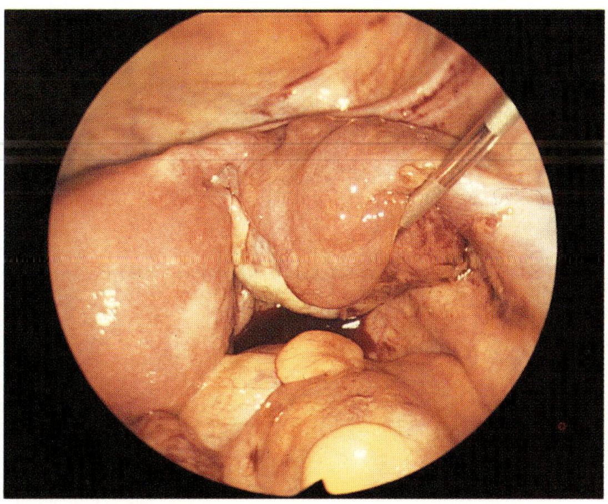

Case 2.3

A 19-year-old female with fever and RLQ peritonitis. The WBC count was 14,000 with a marked left shift. Pelvic exam was normal. Note the inflamed cecum with normal appearing appendix. The terminal ileum with cock's comb is seen in the foreground without inflammation. Stool

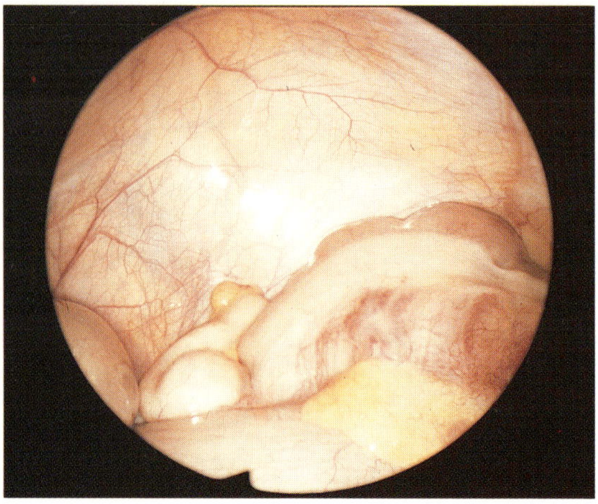

cultures subsequently grew *Salmonella*. Dx: Acute cecal enteritis. In Case 2.3, the clinical picture was identical to that for acute appendicitis, but the history was less typical. Therefore, laparoscopy was carried out before laparotomy. The etiology of the symptoms was clear, and an unnecessary appendectomy was avoided. It is easy to appreciate the closeness of the inflammation in the cecum to the appendix, which explains the difficulty in making the diagnosis.

Case 2.4

A 26-year-old male with fever and RLQ peritonitis. There was a known history of acquired immune deficiency syndrome (AIDS). The WBC count was normal. The palpating probe is seen lifting an acutely inflamed appendix. Note exudate at the tip and base of the appendix. A

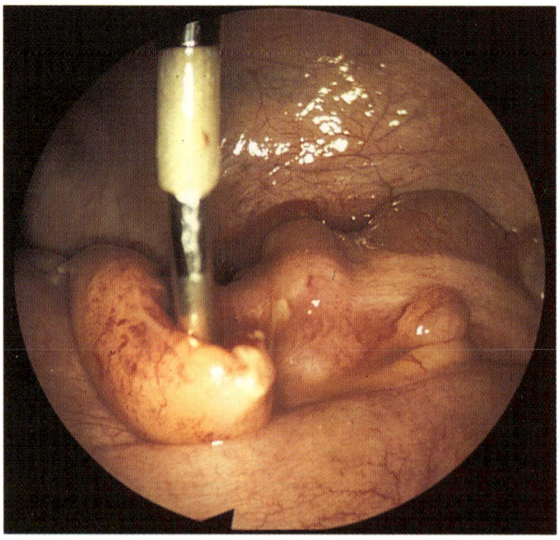

normal loop of small bowel is visible in the foreground. Dx: Acute appendicitis. Case 2.4 demonstrates the findings of acute appendicitis with a normal WBC count. The history of AIDS should alert the surgeon to other infectious processes that can mimic appendicitis. Negative surgical procedures in immunocompromised patients increase morbidity and mortality. Laparoscopy under local anesthesia is ideal in exactly this setting.

Case 2.5

A 39-year-old female with fever and RLQ peritonitis. Pelvic exam was unremarkable. The WBC count was 10,300 without a left shift. Laparoscopic view of blood in the right peritoneal gutter is shown. A normal appendix is clearly seen surrounded by normal mesoappendiceal fat. Dx: Ruptured corpus luteal cyst with hemorrhage. Aspiration of the blood through a second puncture site relieved the pain. Case 2.5 again demonstrates a common diagnostic problem for the surgeon. Ovulatory bleeding is usually easily differentiated from appendicitis. Occasionally, it is very difficult to tell the difference with reasonable certainty, when the bleeding ascends the right peritoneal gutter. Laparoscopy will easily differentiate.

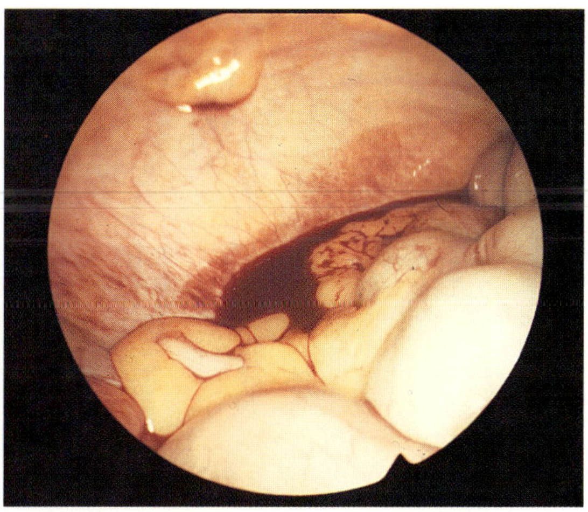

Case 2.6

A 32-year-old female with fever and RLQ peritonitis. The WBC count was 15,000 with a marked left shift. Laparoscopic view of cecal enteritis with inflammation only on the the medial wall of the cecum. The appendix was normal. Dx: Cecal enteritis. The stool cultures subsequently grew *Yersinia* species. Case 2.6 illustrates another common reason for

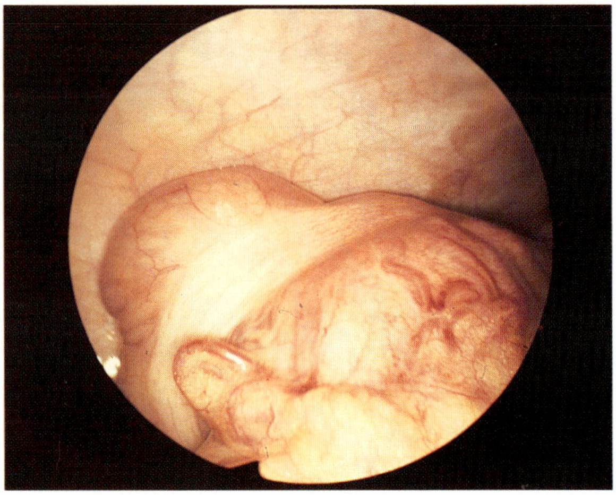

negative appendectomies. *Yersinia* is frequently the culprit in mimicking acute appendicitis, especially in younger age groups. The reason for the difficulty in differentiating appendicitis from cecal and ascending colon enteritis is clearly demonstrated in this laparoscopic picture. When the inflammatory process occurs near the appendix, it may be impossible to tell the difference on clinical findings alone. Laparoscopy is ideal in this setting.

Case 2.7

A 25-year-old male with fever and RLQ peritonitis. The patient had known idiopathic thrombocytopenic purpura with a platelet count of

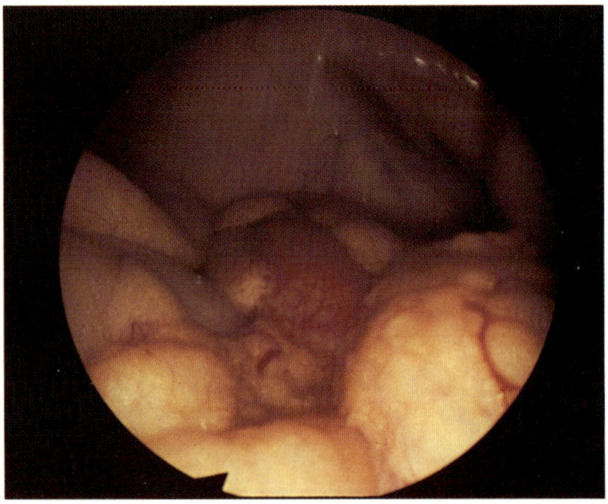

50,000 and AIDS. The WBS was normal. Abdominal sonogram was negative for retroperitoneal hematoma. Laparoscopic view of an inflamed, swollen appendix. A normal loop of small bowel is seen at the left for comparison. The omentum is to the right. Dx: Acute appendicitis. Case 2.7 demonstrates another high-risk patient. Although the differential diagnosis of RLQ pain is less a problem in males than females, it is certainly just as important, especially in the high-risk patient. The patient underwent an uncomplicated appendectomy.

Case 2.8

A 19-year-old female with 7-hr history of RLQ pain without fever or elevated WBC count. Note the increased vascularity of the appendix, as compared to that of the sera of the surrounding bowel loops. Dx: Early acute appendicitis. Case 2.8 shows that elevation of the WBC count or fever are not necessarily features of early acute appendicitis. While it is true that this was an early pickup, it does point to the accuracy of laparoscopy in the diagnosis of acute RLQ pain.

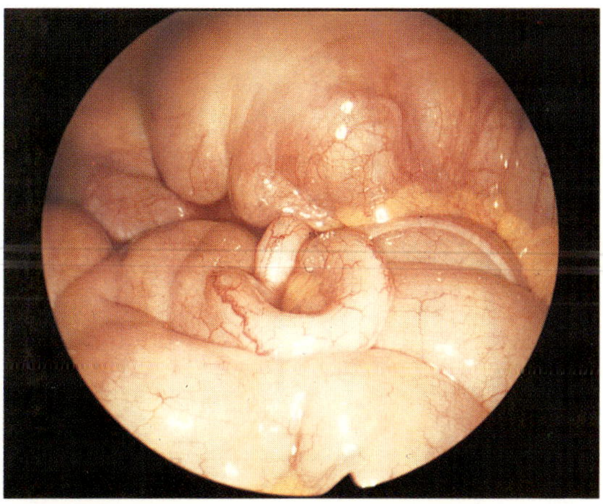

Case 2.9

A 45-year-old female with acute RLQ pain without fever or leukocytosis. Note exudate on the cecum with edema of the right colon parietal peritoneal attachments. The appendix could not be visualized. Case 2.9 again demonstrates acute appendicitis (retrocecal) without elevation of the WBC count or fever.

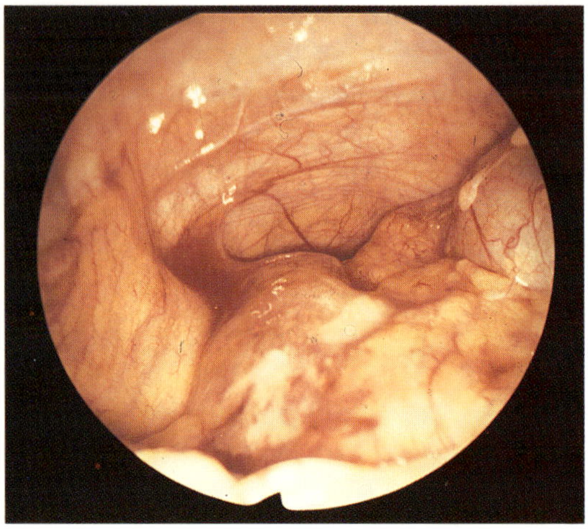

Case 2.10

A 42-year-old female with bilateral lower peritonitis, 24,000 WBC count with marked left shift, fever, and mild diarrhea. Laparoscopic view of severe small bowel inflammation with intense hyperemia and petechia of the serosa. Approximately 6 feet of the proximal ileum were involved. The appendix and terminal ileum were normal, which can be seen on the right. The uterus and right fallopian tube are seen in the background. Dx: Acute enteritis. Case 2.10 is interesting in that the clinical diagnosis was an acute abdomen. The patient's lower abdominal wall was rigid. The laparoscopy was performed to help with proper laparotomy incision placement, as the diagnosis was not at all clear. Much to the author's surprise, a nonsurgical cause was found. Cultures were negative, and the patient improved dramatically in the next 24 hours.

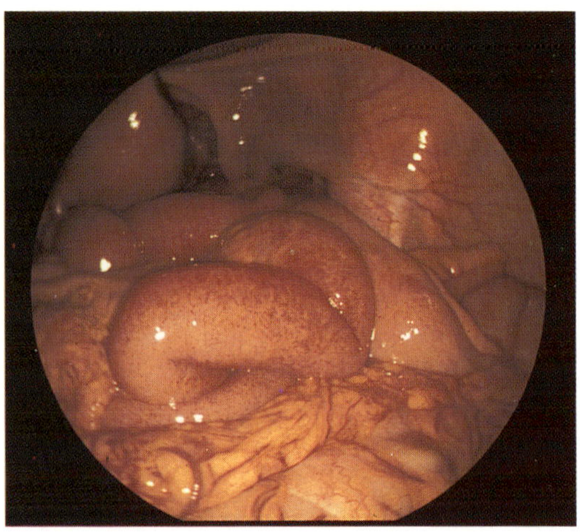

Discussion

In all of the above cases, a clear-cut diagnosis of acute right lower quadrant pain was not possible based on the history, physical examination, laboratory data, or radiographs. If the diagnosis of appendicitis was clear, laparoscopy was not undertaken. In several of these cases, there were associated medical problems that put them at high risk for general anesthesia or for a negative exploration. Most of the patients underwent laparoscopy with local anesthesia accompanied by mild intravenous sedation. In each of these cases, laparoscopy was definitive.

Retrocecal appendicitis may be difficult to diagnose from clinical data, and it also presents some difficulties from a laparoscopic point of view as well. Case 2.9 illustrates the common findings in retroperitoneal inflammation with edema and hyperemia of the parietal peritoneum. Sometimes the wall of the cecum may be thickened, which can be appreciated with the second puncture probe. But in early cases, these dramatic changes are absent. Therefore, if the primary indication for laparoscopy is the diagnosis of acute RLQ pain and the appendix cannot be visualized, a formal exploration of the appendix is warranted. In the author's experience, this has been the cause of the sole negative appendectomy in the last 8 years.

RIGHT UPPER QUADRANT PAIN

Case 2.11

A 23-year-old female with right upper quadrant (RUQ) peritonitis. Sonogram and pelvic examination were normal. Note significant amount of hemorrhage on surface of liver capsule. Normal gallbladder clearly seen. Gynecological organs and pelvis demonstrate no abnormalities. No liver tumor or history of trauma. Dx: Hemoperitoneum,

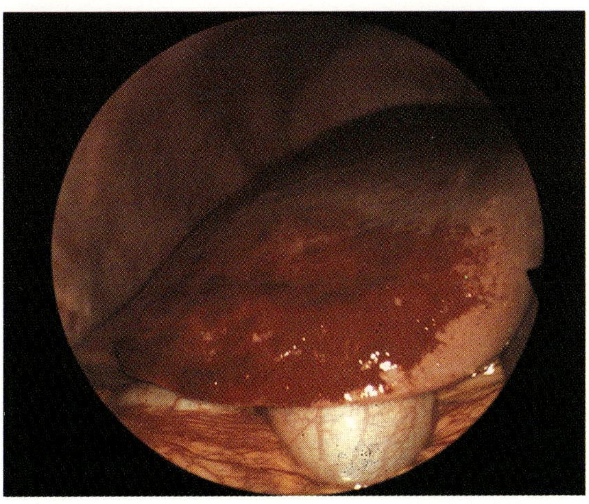

etiology unknown. Case 2.11 clearly illustrates the advantage of laparoscopy. This patient's physical examination was remarkable for peritoneal findings in the RUQ. However, none of the laboratory or radiological data confirmed an inflammatory disease. Although the etiology was never elucidated, the sparing of a laparotomy for diagnosis was accomplished. The patient recovered with observation only. Subsequent workup was negative.

Case 2.12

A 55-year-old female with RUQ peritonitis. The temperature and WBC counts were normal. Sonogram showed gallstones but without edema of the gallbladder. The HIDA scan was normal. Laparoscopic view of exudate over the medial aspect of the gallbladder and medial segment of the left lobe of the liver. There were smaller exudative deposits on the superior aspect of liver capsule and right hemidiaphragm. Dx: Acute retroileal appendicitis with "metastatic" exudate. Appendicitis can present as RUQ peritonitis without the usual RLQ peritoneal findings. Case 2.12 shows the exudative process in the RUQ of this case of ruptured retroileal appendicitis. The physical findings in the RLQ were minimal. Laparoscopy was helpful in planning a proper RLQ incision.

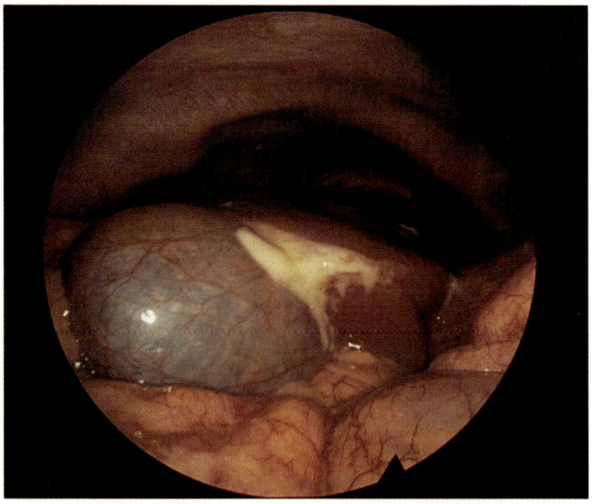

Case 2.13*A* and *B*

A 50-year-old male presented with a 10-day history of RUQ pain, fever, and weight loss. The CT scan in Figure 2.13**A** demonstrates a hypodense area in the right lobe of the liver. The laparoscopic view (Fig. 2.13**B**) revealed acute cholecystitis with pericholecystic abscess and perforation

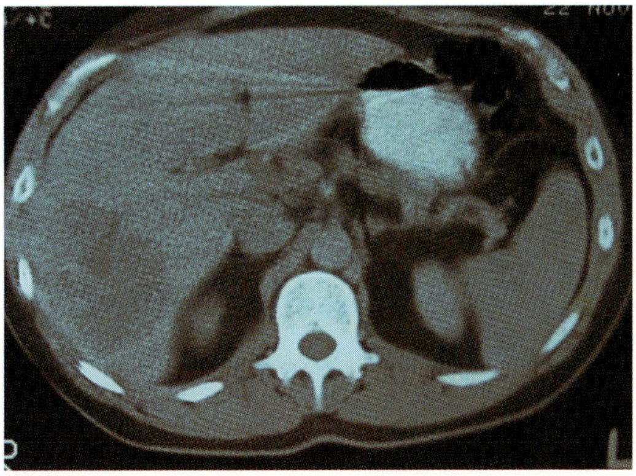

A

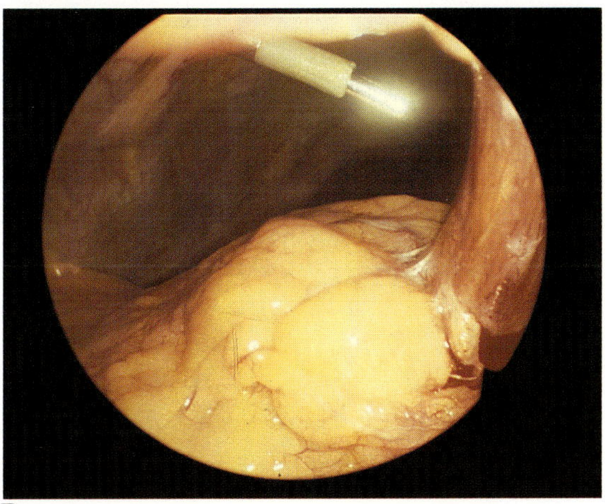

B

into the liver. Omental adhesions to the gallbladder and round ligament can be seen below palpating probe. The results of CT scan in case 2.13 were consistent with those of tumor. The history and physical exam were more consistent with those of an inflammatory process. A thorough GI evaluation was negative. Laparoscopy was undertaken to define further the extent of disease and to determine potentially any other metastatic disease that would preclude laparotomy. Once the omental adhesions were taken down with the palpating probe, the true nature of the problem became obvious, and an uneventful cholecystectomy and drainage of abscess were performed.

Case 2.14

An 82-year-old female presented with RUQ pain, fever, and an epigastric mass. The patient had severe coronary artery disease. A sonogram demonstrated a thickened gallbladder without calculi, and a HIDA scan

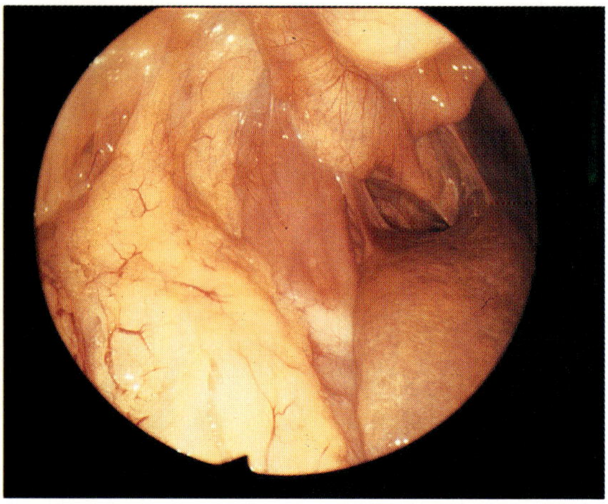

was normal. CT scan showed a 'tumor mass'' in the RUQ separate from the liver. Laparoscopic view shows omental adhesions and duodenum pulled into an inflammatory mass in the RUQ. Round ligament is at the superior right aspect of picture. Left lobe of the liver is normal. Dx: Subacute acalculous cholecystitis. Laparoscopy was undertaken in case 2.14, as the patient was thought to have a "malignant" process and directed biopsy was to be performed. However, the laparoscopic appearance was that of an inflammatory process. An uneventful cholecystectomy was performed.

Discussion

RUQ pain can be difficult to diagnose, although with the advent of sonography and CT scanning it is much less a problem. Nevertheless, there is a use for laparoscopy in the occasional patient in whom these tests are unrewarding. I have found the major indication to be in the differential diagnosis of malignant versus benign disease. Case 2.14 is a good example. If a malignant process had been found laparoscopically, no further intervention would have been recommended because of her associated medical problems. Case 2.11 involved a very difficult clinical problem in which the laparoscopy truly negated the need for a laparotomy. Laparoscopy is not recommended in straightforward cases in which a laparotomy is clearly indicated.

Case 2.15*A–C*

A 27-year-old male presented with acute epigastric and right upper quadrant pain. He was afebrile, and all the laboratory data were normal. Physical examination revealed marked epigastric and right of midline peritonitis. Noninvasive scanning was normal. Laparoscopic view of the upper abdominal cavity with omentum adhered to the midline (Fig.

2.15**A**). The liver is visible in the background as is the gallbladder faintly. Figure 2.15**B** shows the omentum partially dissected away from the abdominal wall. An area of linear infarction is seen with a small amount of exudate present. The round ligament is to the immediate right of the omentum. Figure 2.15**C** demonstrates the omentum dissected off completely, and now lying in its normal position. The liver is clearly visible. The area of infarction is just seen at the bottom of the picture. Dx: Infarcted omentum. Laparoscopy was definitive regarding this patient's diagnosis. The small area of infarction was left in place with marked improvement in the symptoms. However, over the next month, the patient had intermittent epigastric pain not associated with peritoneal findings. The patient underwent an elective omentectomy with complete regression of the pain. The laparoscopy was performed under local anesthesia.

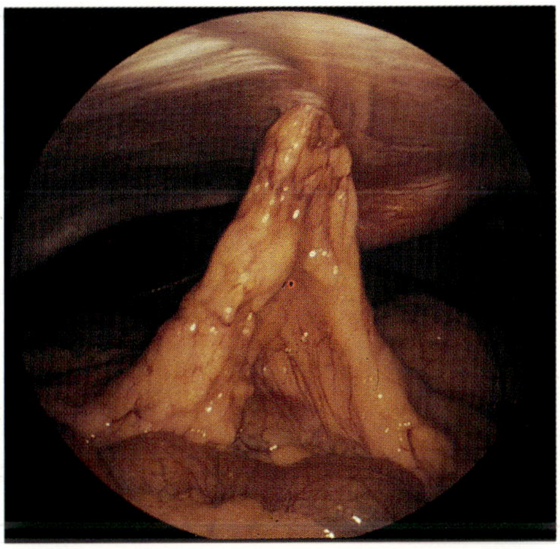

A

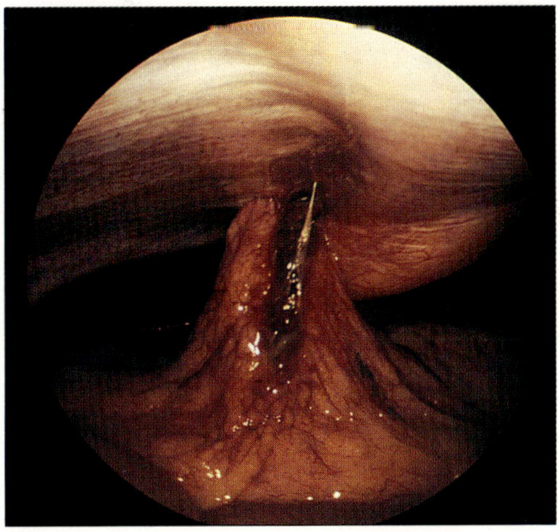

B

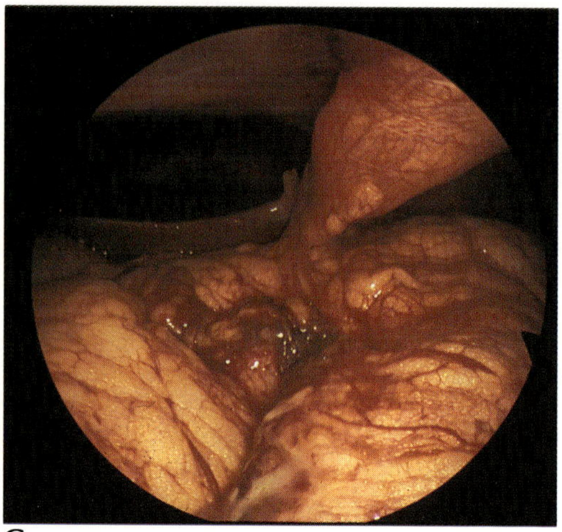

C

Case 2.16

A 36-year-old female presented with right upper quadrant peritoneal findings. She had a low grade fever and mild leukocytosis. Sonogram and HIDA scans were normal. Laparoscopic view of the right upper quadrant demonstrating exudate over an inflammatory mass. The liver is in the background. Although not shown on this photo, the gallbladder and appendix were visualized and were normal. Dx. Right transverse colon diverticulitis. This patient's diagnosis was not obvious based on the history or physical exam. Laparoscopy was performed under local anesthesia. The diagnosis was confirmed by barium enema and CT scan performed as an outpatient after a one week course of intravenous antibiotics. She has remained asymptomatic.

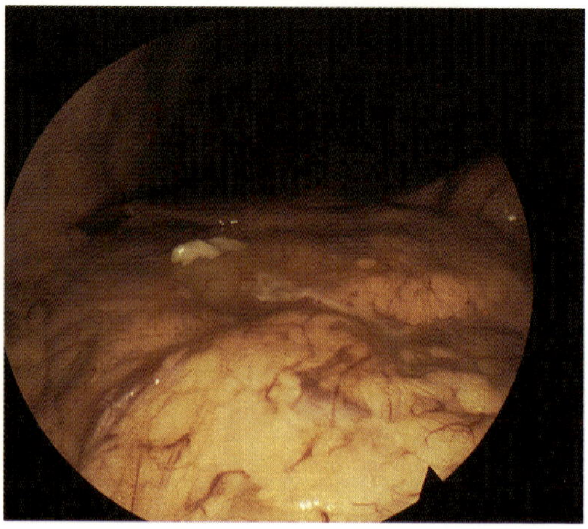

Case 2.17A–C

A 45-year-old female presented with acute right lower quadrant pain. Besides a rigid RLQ, all other lab tests, radiographs, and sonogram were normal. The patient was status post appendectomy and hysterectomy. Both ovaries were still in place. Laparoscopic view of the right lower quadrant showing an inflamed omentum adhered to the parietal peritoneum (Fig. 2.17**A**). Figure 2.17**B** demonstrates probe dissection of the omentum off the peritoneal surface. Note the extreme erythema of the parietal surface. The omentum is still partially attached to the peritoneum. Figure 2.17**C** illustrates the infarcted omentum now moved to just beneath the laparoscopic incision by the suction-coagulator probe. A loop of ileum is visible just next to the infarction. The preoperative diagnosis was either infarcted omentum or ruptured ovarian cyst.

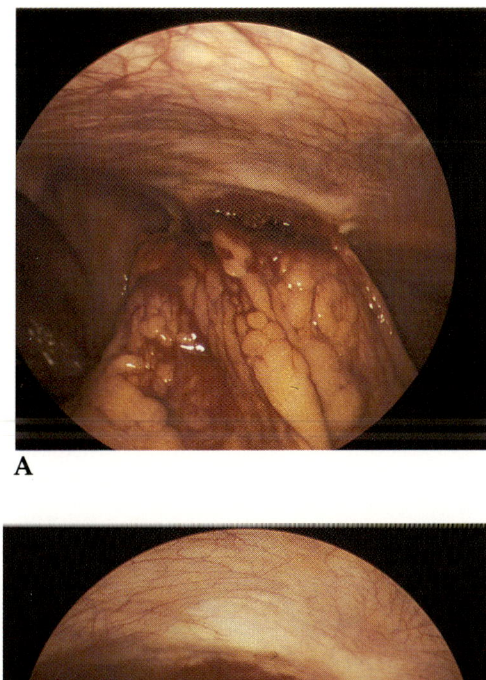

A

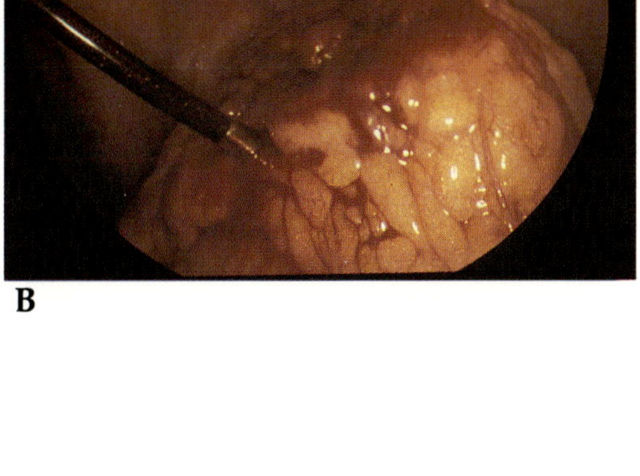

B

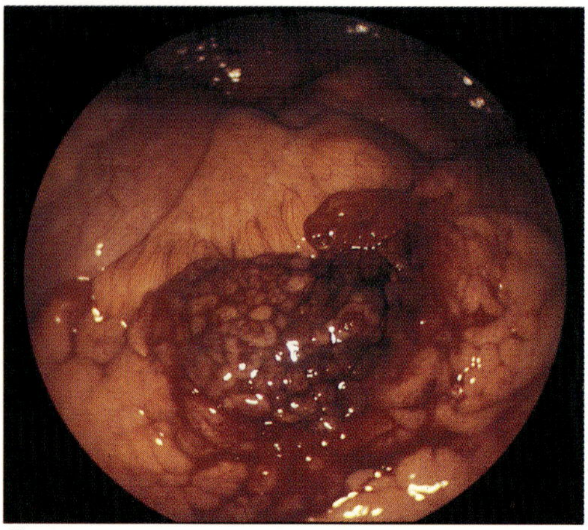

C

The laparoscopy was not only diagnostic but also allowed manipulation of the infarction to directly beneath the laparoscopic puncture wound. This allowed a slight extension of the original 1-cm incision to extract the infarcted omentum, which the patient appreciated from a cosmetic point of view. Total hospital stay was 2 days.

CHRONIC ABDOMINAL PAIN

Chronic recurrent abdominal pain syndromes are frequently frustrating experiences for patient and surgeon alike. All patients undergo extensive testing that includes multiple contrast radiographs, endoscopies, sonograms, and CT scans. Many of these tests are a repeated search for a cause. The economic cost is enormous. In the author's experience, 40% have a history of at least one previous laparotomy before the onset of the pain. Not surprisingly, adhesions are then assumed to be the cause of the pain. Laparoscopy will define the etiology in 55% of these difficult patients. It is most important to perform the laparoscopy under local anesthesia so that the patient can help localize the pain upon movement of the abdominal viscera. In some cases, therapeutic manipulations via the laparoscope will be definitive. (See Chapter 6; Therapeutic Laparoscopy.)

Case 2.18

A 24-year-old female with multiple episodes of RLQ pain over a 2-year-period. She had one febrile event 1 year earlier and normal lab values. Note hyperemia of the appendix with adhesions fixing the appendix to the iliac fossa. The mesoappendix is thickened. The cecum is pulled upward by the palpating probe. Dx: Recurrent appendicitis. An appendectomy was performed.

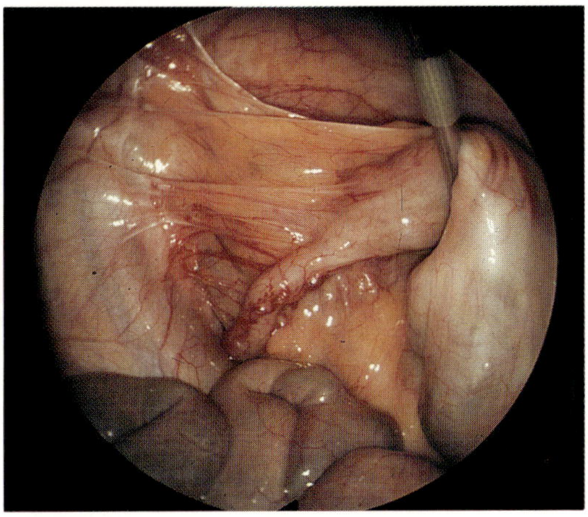

Case 2.19

A 36-year-old female with a 3-year history of intermittent RLQ pain. No fever or abnormal lab values. Note appendix and mesoappendix twisted on itself with shortening of the mesoappendix. Palpating probe is on the cecum. Dx: Chronic recurrent appendicitis. An appendectomy was performed.

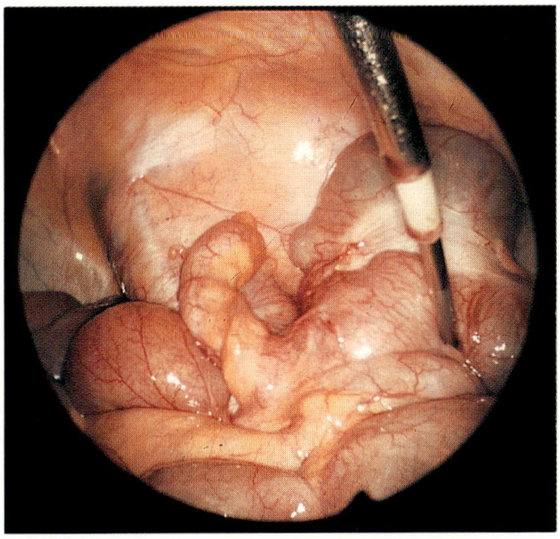

Case 2.20

An 18-year-old male with a 1-year history of recurrent RLQ pain and a history of left-sided ulcerative colitis. There was no fever but mild chronic leukocytosis secondary to prednisone. Mild hyperemia of the appendix with thickening of the mesoappendix was present. Dx: Chronic recurrent appendicitis. An uneventful appendectomy was performed.

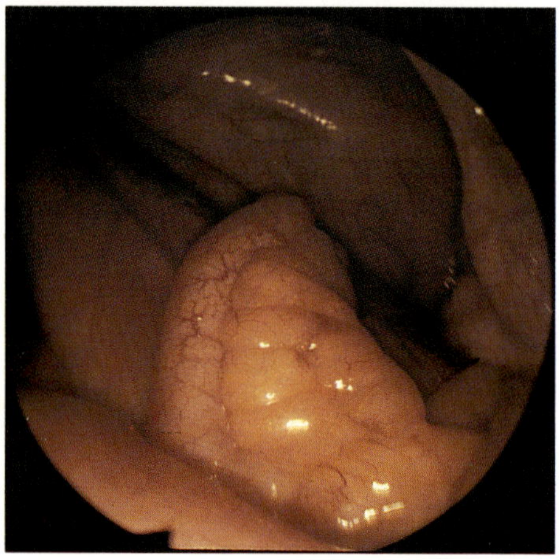

Case 2.21

An 18-year-old female with known gallstones and atypical recurrent right-sided abdominal pain. No fever or abnormal lab data. Laparoscopy was performed before cholecystectomy. Surprise finding of fecalith in appendix with mild hyperemia of the appendix. Uneventful appendectomy performed. Patient is now 4 years postop with asymptomatic gallstones.

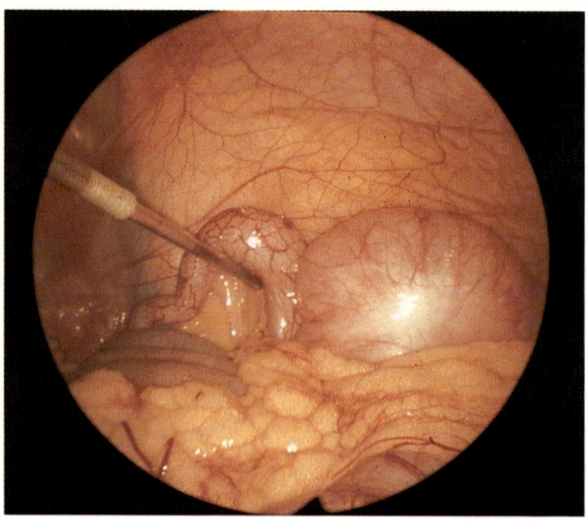

Case 2.22

A 12-year-old male with 1-year history of recurrent pain with one episode of fever. The WBC count was normal. Note hyperemia of the distal portion of the appendix. Dx: Recurrent appendicitis. Uneventful laparoscopic appendectomy was performed. (See chapter 6; Therapeutic Laparoscopy.) Pathology revealed acute mucosal inflammation with severe lymphoid hyperplasia.

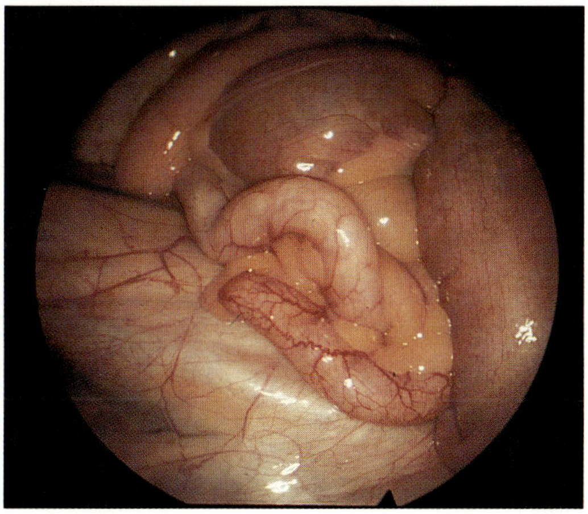

Case 2.23

A 24-year-old male with 2-year history of recurrent episodic RLQ pain. All workups were normal. Laparoscopic view of mucocele of appendix. Normal cecum is in the *background*. Dx: Mucocele of appendix. Pathol-

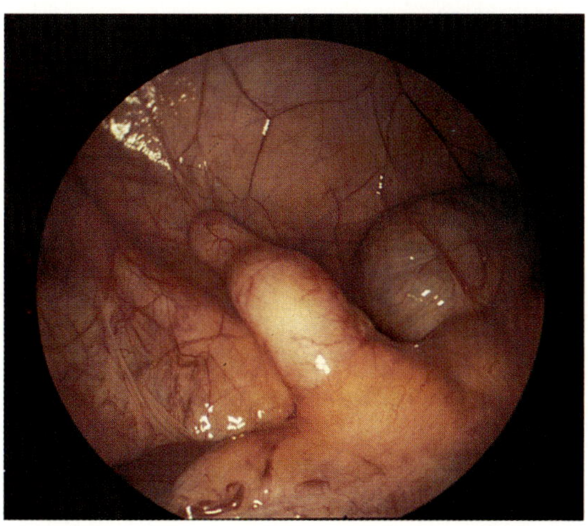

ogy showed severe lymphoid hyperplasia. Although the natural history of acute appendicitis usually requires early appendectomy, resolution with chronic recurrent pain does exist, as noted in cases 2.11 through 2.16. The pathology of each appendix confirmed inflammatory disease. In each patient, the preoperative symptomatology disappeared after the appendectomy. The laparoscope is ideally suited for diagnosis and sometimes for treatment of appendicitis. Laparoscopic appendectomy will be discussed in detail in Chapter 6; Therapeutic Laparoscopy.

Case 2.24

A 33-year-old male with recurrent RLQ pain and occasional diarrhea. UGI and small bowel series were normal. Barium enema with reflux into the terminal ileum was normal. Note the short segment of typical Crohn's disease with creeping of the mesenteric fat and lymphadenopathy in the mesentery. Small bowel Crohn's disease is usually easily diagnosed by barium contrast studies. However, if the terminal ileum is spared, as in this case, the diagnosis can be missed radiologically. A firm diagnosis is necessary before the institution of steroids. Laparoscopy is ideal in this setting, as the distal 5 to 6 feet of ileum are readily visualized with the laparoscope.

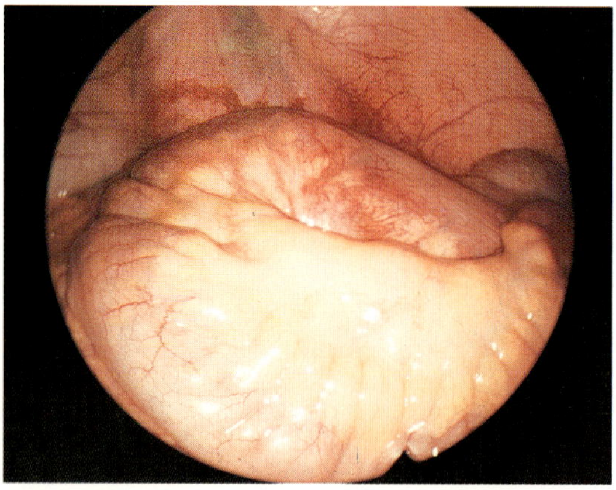

Case 2.25

A 29-year-old female with recurrent RUQ pain. Known past history of pelvic inflammatory disease (PID). Sonography of the abdomen and pelvis were normal. Note the typical violin string adhesions between the anterior capsule of the liver and the diaphragm. Dx: Fitzhugh-Curtis syndrome. Although the presumptive prelaparoscopic diagnosis was Fitzhugh-Curtis syndrome, some symptomatic relief was obtained by laparoscopic lysis of adhesions. It is interesting in that the insufflation of the pneumoperitoneum immediately caused the patient to complain of the same type of pain. It is not clear whether this is secondary to Glisson capsule stretch or pull on the parietal peritoneum of the right hemidiaphragm. There was partial relief of pain immediately after laparoscopic lysis.

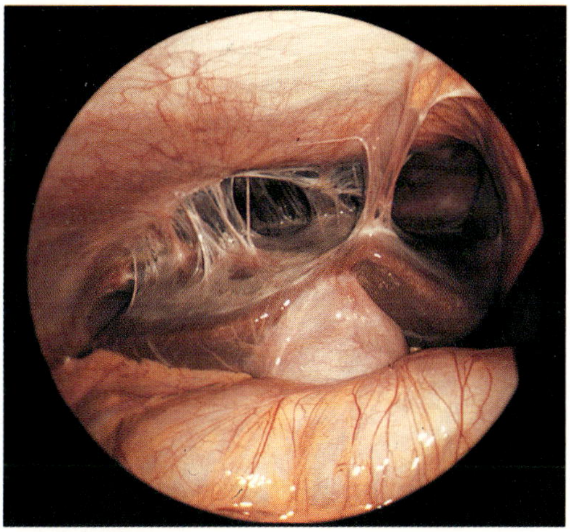

Case 2.26

A 32-year-old female with recurrent RLQ pain. GYN examination prelaparoscopy was felt to be normal. A palpating probe can be seen over the right fallopian tube. Note the swelling in the tube itself. Dx: Hydrosalpinx of the right tube.

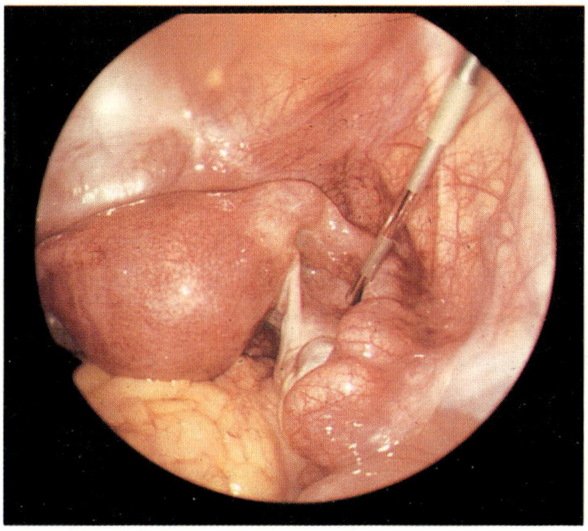

Case 2.27

A 26-year-old female with recurrent RLQ pain. Pelvic exam was normal, and sonography was normal. Laparoscopic view of endometrial implants at the base of the urinary bladder just superior to the broad ligament. Dx: Endometriosis. Gynecological pathology will occasionally be encountered in the evaluation of abdominal pain syndromes. Therefore, it is important to be familiar with gynecological pathology as well. Even though the author limits himself to gastrointestinal laparoscopy, cases 2.26 and 2.27 illustrate well the need for familiarity with normal and pathological gynecology, as examination of the pelvic structures are included in the laparoscopic evaluation of the abdominal cavity. Both of these patients were referred by experienced gynecologists believing the problem was in the gastrointestinal tract.

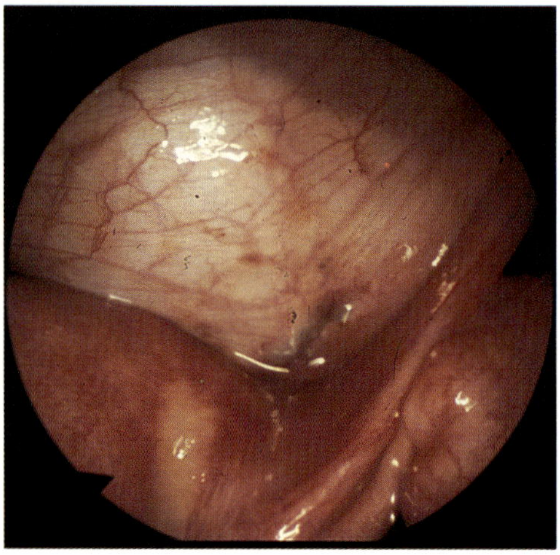

Case 2.28

A 55-year-old female with chronic RUQ pain. The patient had a normal sonogram and oral cholecystogram (OCG). Palpating probe lifting right lobe of the liver superiorly. Note the pale visceral peritoneum over the gallbladder with adhesions to the omentum consistent with some previous inflammatory event. The hepatic flexure of the colon is in the foreground. The cholecystoduodenal attachments are to the right. Dx: Chronic cholecystitis. Cholecystectomy was performed which revealed tiny gallstones. Sonography and oral cholecystography will be accurate in about 98% of the patients with cholelithiasis. In the small group of patients with negative studies and a clinical history consistent with biliary colic, laparoscopy can be helpful. At cholecystectomy, several 2- to 3-mm cholesterol stones were identified. The patient's pain disappeared after the gallbladder was removed. In 1990, a laparoscopic cholecystectomy would be performed.

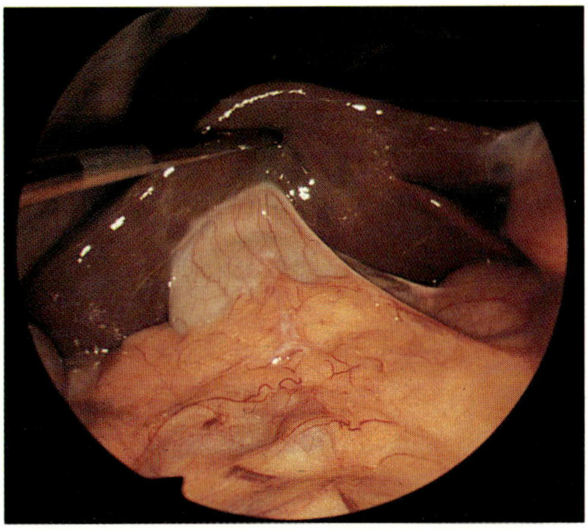

Case 2.29A and B

A 35-year-old female 2 years postappendectomy (for ruptured appendicitis) developed RUQ pain 1 month postop that persisted for 2 years. All radiographs and lab tests were normal. Note the laparoscopic view (Fig. 2.29**A**) of single-band adhesion between the anterior abdominal wall and the omentum with tenting of the stomach (right foreground). Laparoscopic scissors are properly positioned. Figure 2.29**B** demonstrates complete lysis. The right hemidiaphragm can now be seen in the background. This case demonstrates a single-band adhesion between the parietal peritoneum and a viscous causing pinpoint pain. In the author's experience, if a single-band adhesion can be found that, upon traction, reproduces the preop pain, even in the presence of multiple other adhesions, division laparoscopically will dramatically alleviate the complaint. It is imperative that the procedure be accomplished under

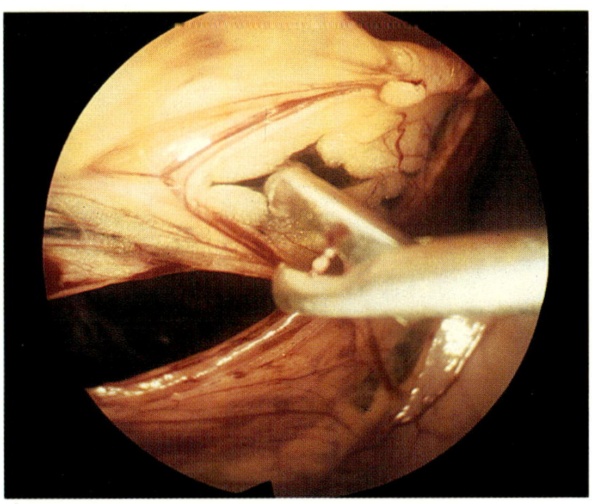

A

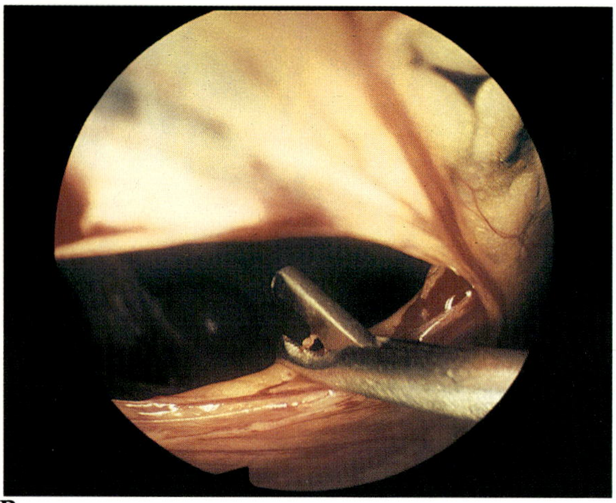

B

local anesthesia so that the patient can help localize the adhesion. If the pain can not be reproduced, lysis should not be undertaken. Small blood vessels such as those demonstrated in the first slide (case 2.29**A**) need not be cauterized before division.

Case 2.30*A–C*

A 26-year-old female 5 years postappendectomy with a 2-year history of recurrent RLQ pain requiring narcotics for relief. Figure 2.30**A** demonstrates a tented up ascending colon with a mobile cecum. The second puncture probe is at left. Figure 2.30**B** shows the proper angle for laparoscopic scissors placement in order to lyse the adhesions. Note the

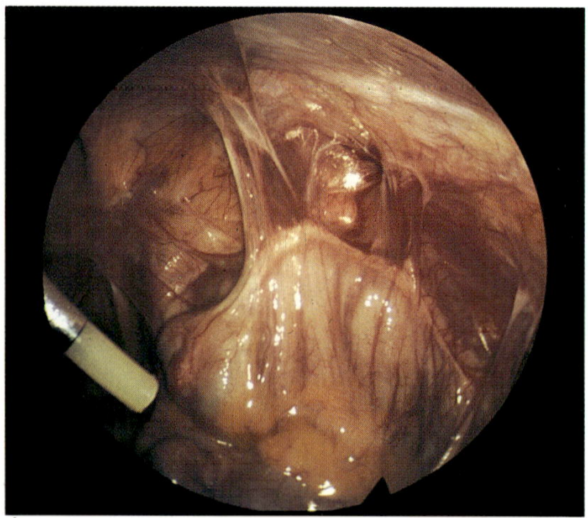

A

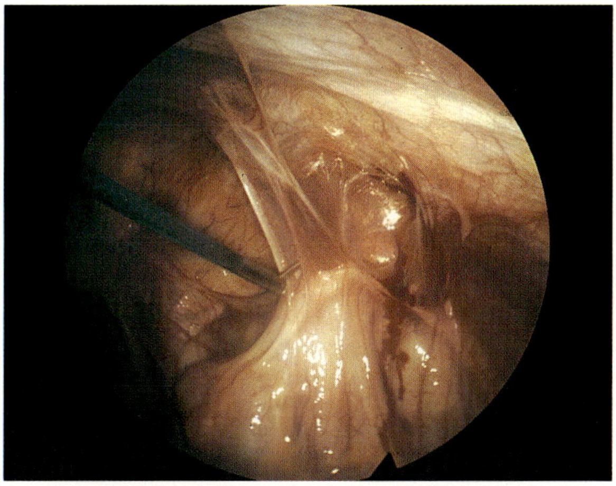

B

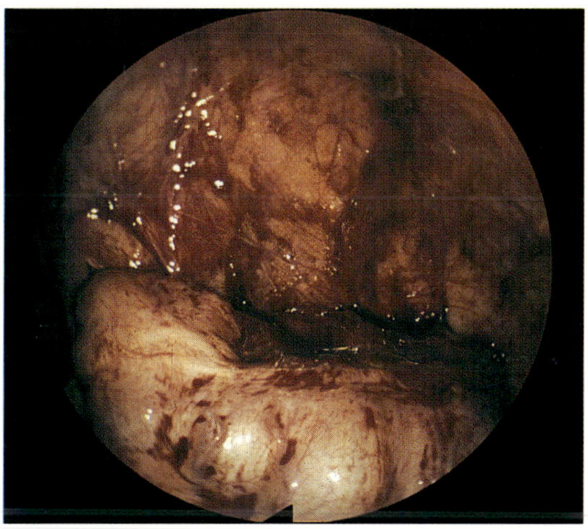

C

clear area between the parietal peritoneum and the colon. In Figure 2.30C, the adhesions have been lysed completely, and the colon has returned to its normal location. The rather dramatic relief of pain was evident on the OR table immediately after the colon was freed. This procedure was performed under local anesthesia with mild intravenous sedation. When attempting lysis, it is important not to pull on the parietal peritoneum, as the patient will experience severe pain. This patient is 3 years postprocedure without pain and is off narcotics.

Case 2.31

A 45-year-old female with recurrent RLQ pain. She had known right pelvic kidney and a small bowel series with questionable Crohn's disease of the ileum. Laparoscopy revealed a normal ileum without evidence of inflammatory disease. The small bowel was displaced by the pelvic kidney. The pain was reproduced by manipulating the pelvic kidney with the second puncture probe. The association of abdominal pain and pelvic kidney is well known. However, the laparoscopy was instrumental in clarifying the small bowel series and in ruling out inflammatory bowel disease. It is important to recognize this entity to avoid an inadvertent biopsy.

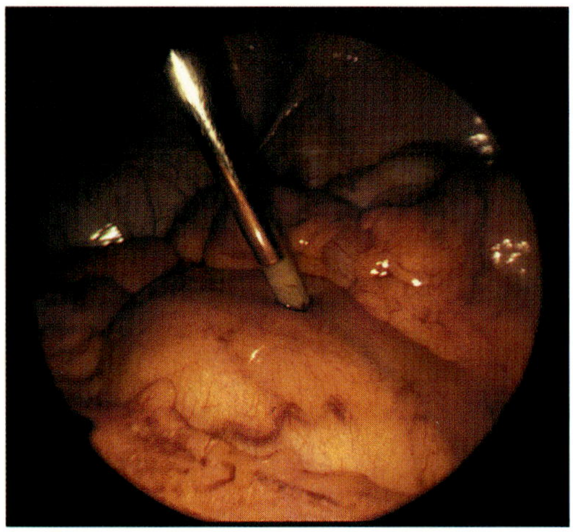

Case 2.32*A–C*

A 34-year-old female presented with a 4-month history of right lower quadrant pain and a 15-pound weight loss. Physical examination revealed a fullness in the right lower quadrant that was mildly tender to palpation. The work-up was negative including barium enema, colonoscopy, CT scan, small bowel series, and all lab data. The patient was 15 years status post appendectomy. Laparoscopic view of the right lower quadrant showing a segment of pneumotosis intestinalis involving a short segment of the ascending colon (Fig. 2.32**A**). The omentum is covering part of the segment, and the air cysts are visible beneath it. Figure 2.32**B** is a closer view of the lateral aspect of the ascending colon. The palpating probe demonstrated this to be very firm on manipulation. Figure 2.32**C** illustrates a close-up of the tiny air sacs present. There is a small area of erythema clearly seen on the colonic wall. Dx: Segmental pneumotosis intestinalis.

This patient was treated with hyperbaric oxygen therapy with dramatic worsening of the pain. Her WBC remained normal. Three weeks after the diagnosis was confirmed by laparoscopy, she underwent an uneventful partial colon resection of the involved ascending colon. Pathology confirmed the diagnosis, and the patient has remained asymptomatic. The right lower quadrant fullness disappeared.

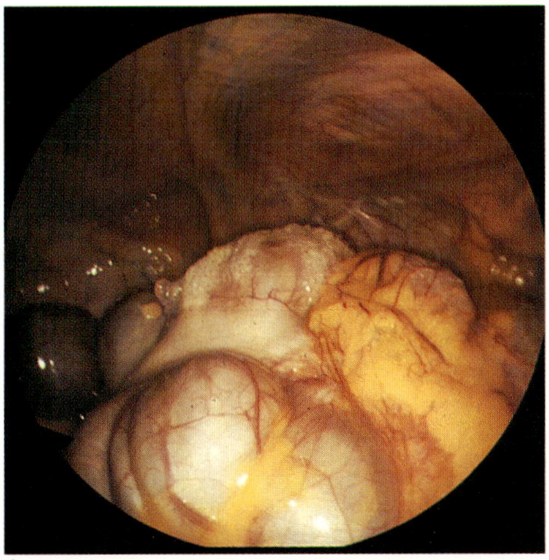

A

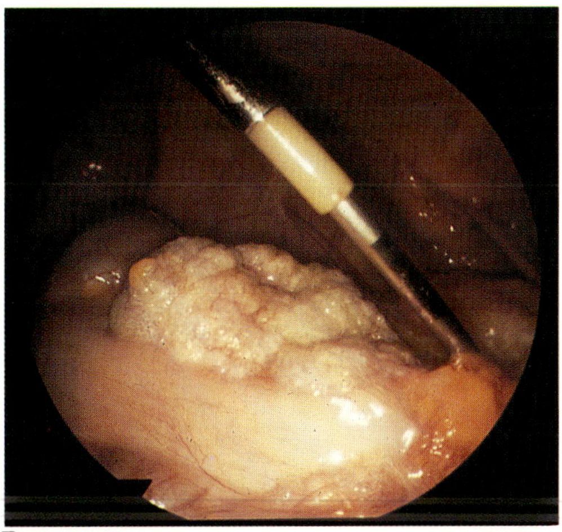

B

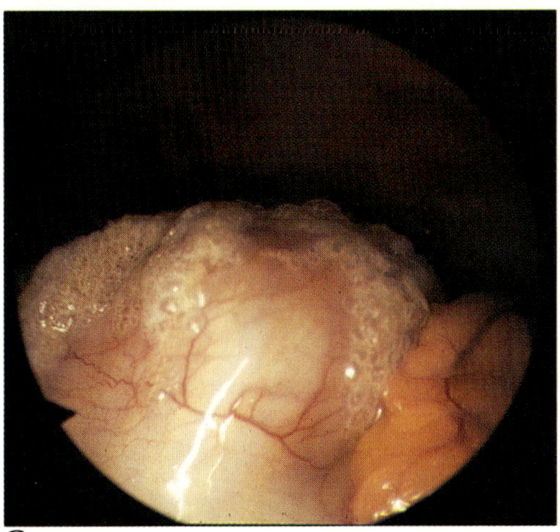

C

3

ABDOMINAL MASSES

The general surgeon is frequently consulted in the evaluation of abdominal masses. Even though sophisticated scanning procedures will almost always anatomically define abdominal masses, direct visualization via laparoscopy affords the surgeon further information regarding its nature. Not all abdominal masses are amenable or desirable for resection. Directed laparoscopic biopsy can easily be accomplished, providing a histological diagnosis. In malignant disease, other metastatic deposits not appreciated on preoperative scans are sometimes found, which may preclude the need for formal laparotomy. This is especially helpful in the high-risk medical patient in whom a negative laparotomy would produce significant morbidity. It is common to perform the laparoscopy immediately before laparotomy so that no delay in hospitalization occurs.

Retroperitoneal masses can also be approached laparoscopically. If the mass is palpable or there is displacement of viscera on preoperative contrast studies, in the author's experience, most will be seen laparoscopically. Therefore, directed biopsy can obtain adequate tissue for histology. In the cases of non-Hodgkin's lymphoma, a positive biopsy will negate the need for laparotomy. This has been the experience in

85% of the cases. The overall diagnostic accuracy of directed laparoscopic biopsy is greater than 95% in all intraabdominal masses.

Case 3.1*A* and *B*

An 89-year-old female presented with a palpable epigastric mass. Sonogram and CT scans were consistent with the presence of a pseudocyst of the pancreas. Because of her severe coronary artery disease, laparoscopy was performed before laparotomy. Figure 3.1**A** demonstrates a large, partially necrotic tumor originating out of the lesser sac pushing the stomach laterally and inferiorly. The edge of the lateral segment of the left lobe of the liver is elevated and seen on the far left. Directed biopsy with the lancet-shaped biopsy forceps into an area away from the nectosis was easily accomplished (Fig. 3.1**B**). A high degree of vascularity was evident. Dx: Spindle cell sarcoma. Because of the pa-

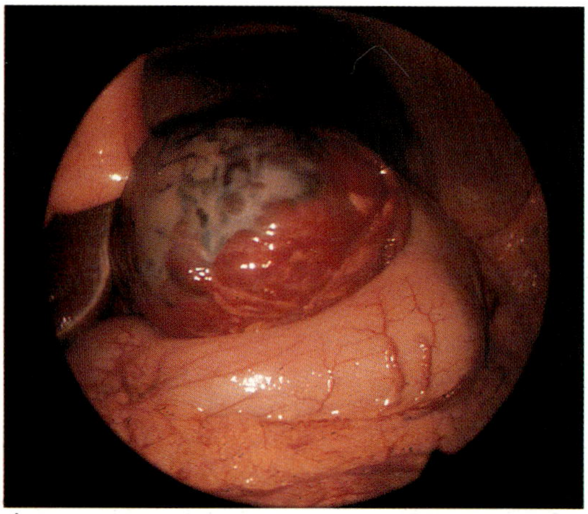

A

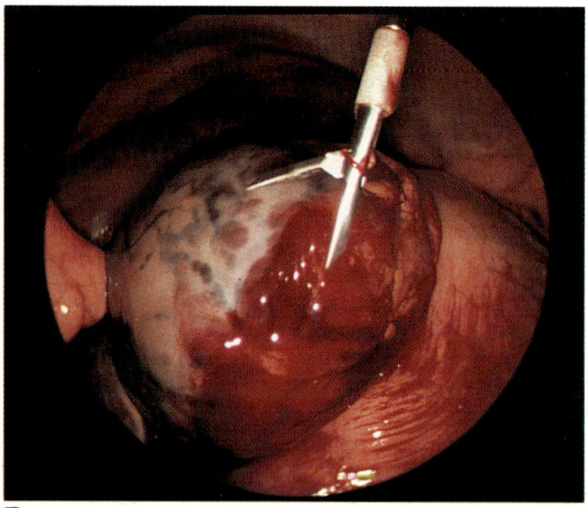

B

tient's advanced age and associated medical problems, resection was not performed. Percutaneous biopsy would have been risky in this highly vascular tumor. Penetration into the necrotic area would likely have resulted in peritonitis. Directed biopsy was safe and yielded the diagnosis.

Case 3.2

A 75-year-old female with back pain underwent CT scanning that showed an abdominal mass. CT scan was read as, most likely, a mesenteric cyst. Laparoscopy demonstrated a partially cystic mass originating from the greater curvature of the stomach. Palpating probe on tumor defines its point of origin. Immediate laparotomy was performed. Dx: Leiomyoma. Laparoscopy was undertaken on the mistaken diagnosis of an asymptomatic cyst. The laparoscopic plan was to aspirate and open a window from the cyst to the peritoneal cavity. Proper diagnosis was made at laparoscopy.

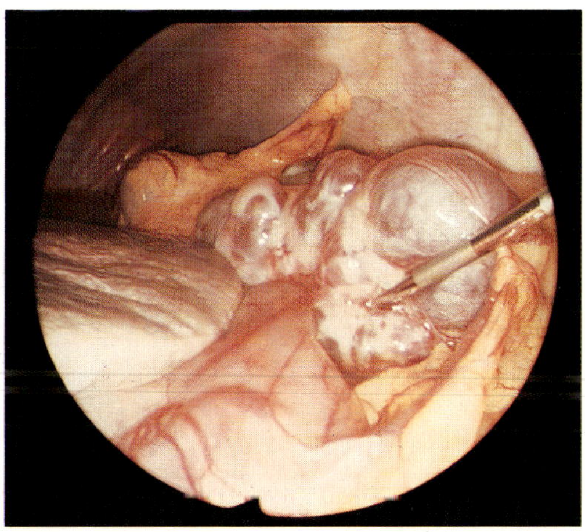

Case 3.3

A 54-year-old female 2 years post left hemicolectomy for adenocarcinoma of the colon. A palpable right lower quadrant (RLQ) mass was present. CT scan showed mass thought to be in the omentum. Laparoscopic view of a large metastatic lesion in the right ovary. Biopsy revealed adenocarcinoma of colonic origin. Dx: Krukenberg tumor. The laparoscopy was undertaken to directly biopsy the mass and to prove the existence of widespread disease, which would preclude laparotomy. However, laparoscopy demonstrated no other metastatic disease, and, therefore, bilateral oophorectomy was undertaken. This patient is now 5 years postop without evidence of disease.

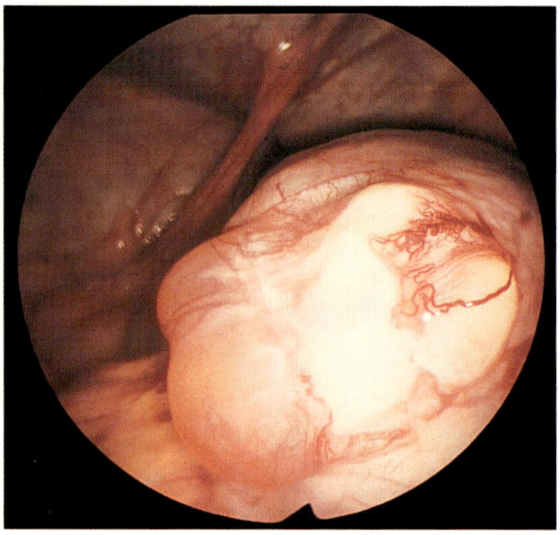

Case 3.4*A* and *B*

An 85-year-old male with right upper quadrant (RUQ) mass. CT scan showed mass confined to the RUQ. Percutaneous needle aspiration was nondiagnostic. Laparoscopy revealed extensive tumor with metastatic parietal peritoneal deposits as well (Fig. 3.4**A**). The round ligament is to the right, and a loop of small bowel is in the foreground. Figure 3.4**B** demonstrates separate tumor growth into the abdominal wall not appreciated on the CT scan. Directed biopsy was easily accomplished. Dx: Colloid adenocarcinoma. Primary unknown. This patient demonstrates well the additional information laparoscopy can obtain for the surgeon. Unresectability was shown quite clearly. As there was nothing to palliate clinically, laparotomy was not undertaken.

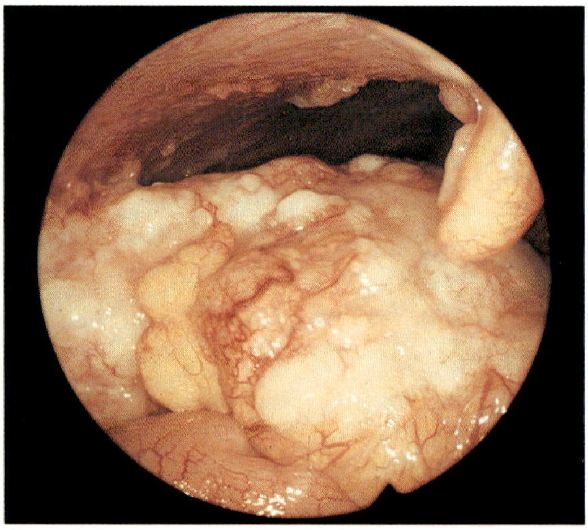

A

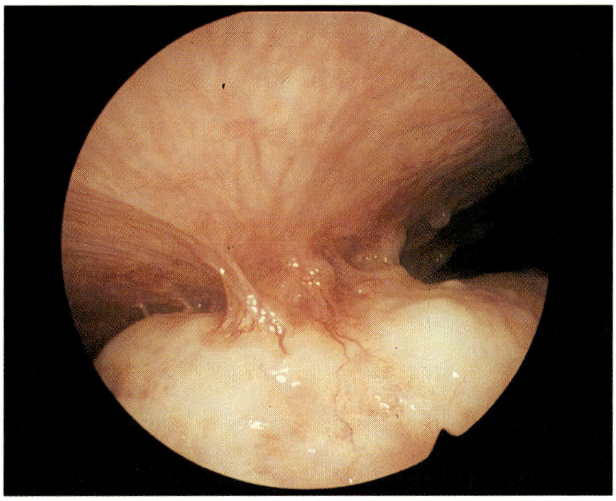

B

Case 3.5*A* and *B*

A 34-year-old female with multiple palpable abdominal masses and weight loss. The CT scan (Fig. 3.5**A**) demonstrated multiple intraabdominal and retroperitoneal masses, some with necrosis. Laparoscopy (Fig. 3.5**B**) revealed a large retroperitoneal tumor mass pushing the small bowel laterally and lifting the transverse colon anteriorly. The small bowel is in the background, and the transverse colon is to the right. Dx: Ganglioneuroma. Tumors that originate in the retroperitoneum but project into the greater sac should be considered intraabdominal from a laparoscopic point of view. They are usually accessible for directed biopsy under laparoscopic control. In this case, the biopsy revealed a "benign" tumor, and as the patient was asymptomatic, no further therapy was instituted. The patient remains without symptoms now 3 years post-procedure.

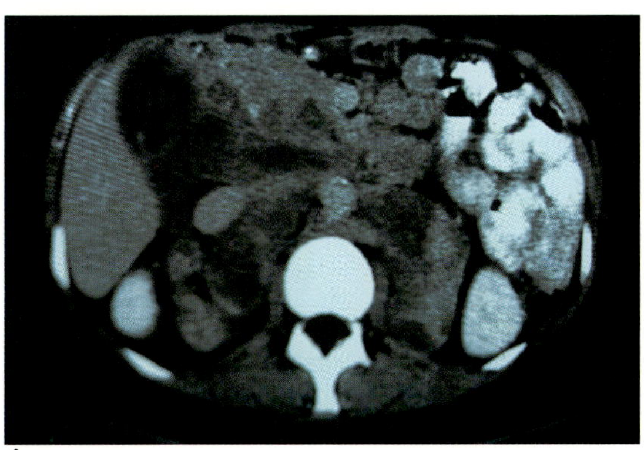

A

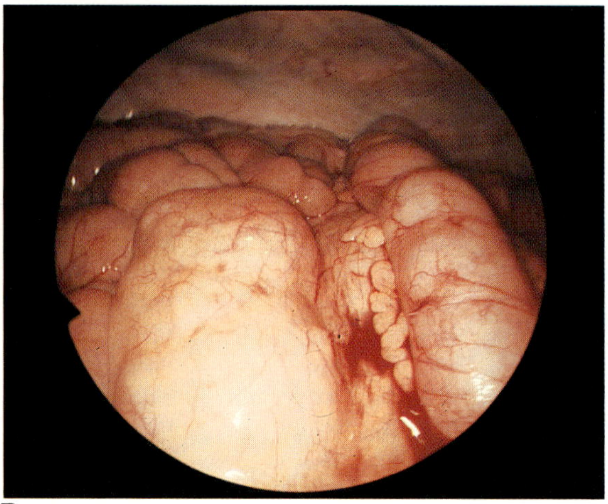

B

Case 3.6*A* and *B*

A 46-year-old male presented with fevers and a palpable RLQ mass. Figure 3.6**A** is the CT scan that demonstrates the mass with areas of

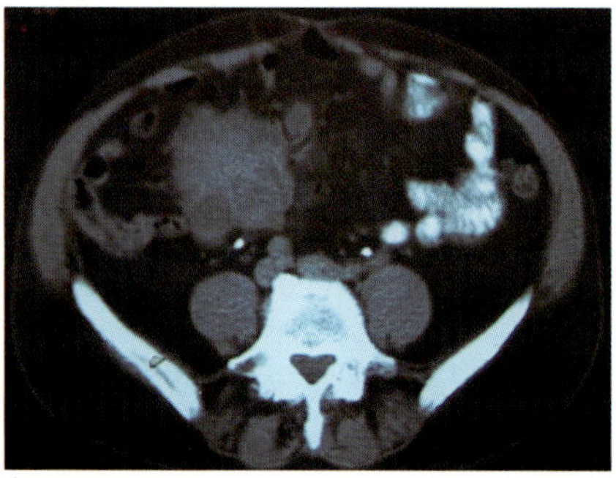

A

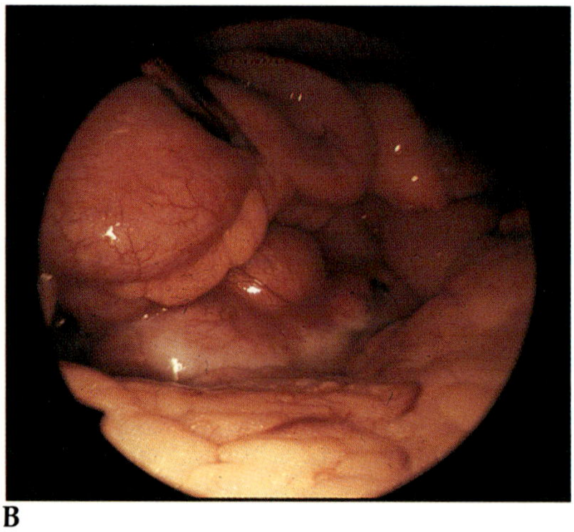

B

necrosis just ventral to the right ureter. Infiltration of the small bowel mesentery should be noted. Figure 3.6**B** reveals the RLQ with the 3-mm palpating probe pushing the small bowel inferiorly. The omentum is in the foreground. A partially necrotic tumor is clearly seen. Directed biopsy was performed. Dx: Non-Hodgkin's lymphoma.

Case 3.7*A* and *B*

A 65-year-old male 2 years postcholecystectomy with fever and weight loss. CT scan demonstrates peripancreatic lymphadenopathy underneath the left lobe of the liver (Fig. 3.7**A**). Metal clip artifact is present at the gallbladder fossa. Laparoscopy showed enlarged lymph glands protruding through the lesser sac (Fig. 3.7**B**). Postsurgical adhesion and hepatic steatosis are incidental findings. Biopsy demonstrated malignant lymphoma.

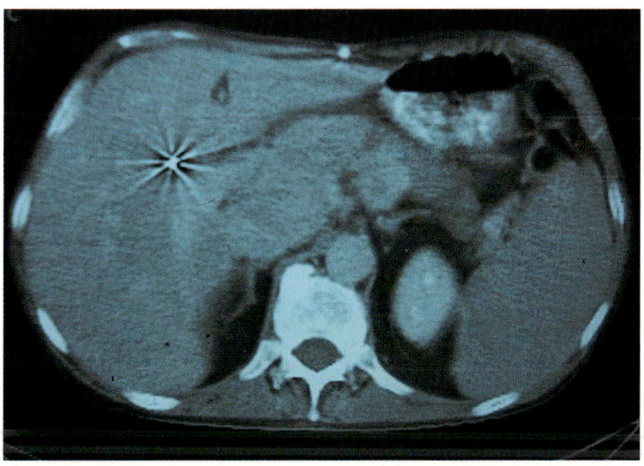

A

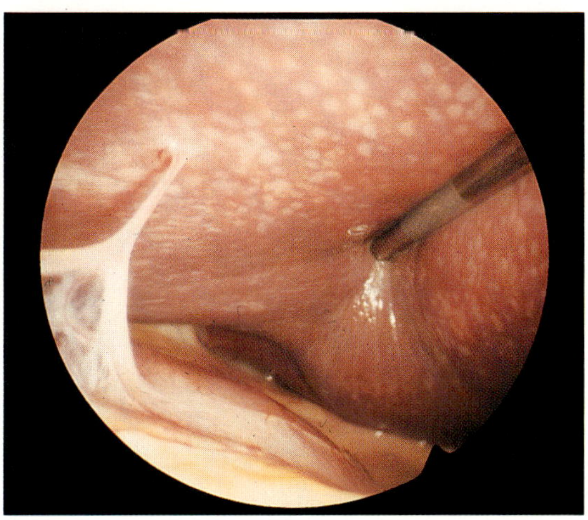

B

Case 3.8*A* and *B*

A 52-year-old male with recent weight loss, fevers, and a palpable epigastric mass. CT scan demonstrated massive retroperitoneal adenopathy. Sonographic guided aspiration was nondiagnostic. Laparoscopic view of multiple enlarged retroperitoneal lymph nodes displacing the omentum superiorly and the small bowel laterally and inferiorly (Fig. 3.8**A**). Biopsy site shows clot (Fig. 3.8**B**). Dx: Non-Hodgkin's lymphoma.

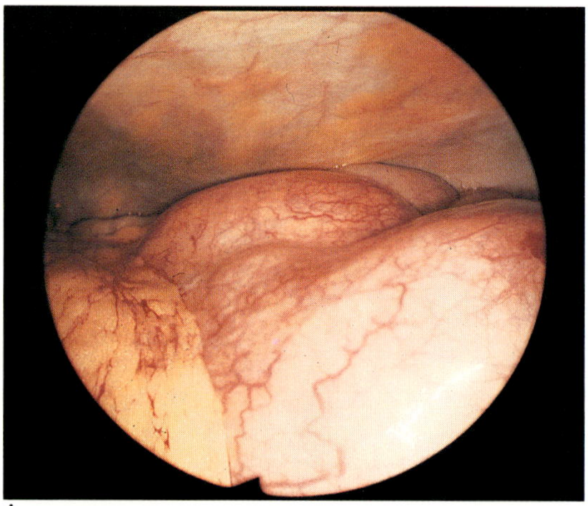

A

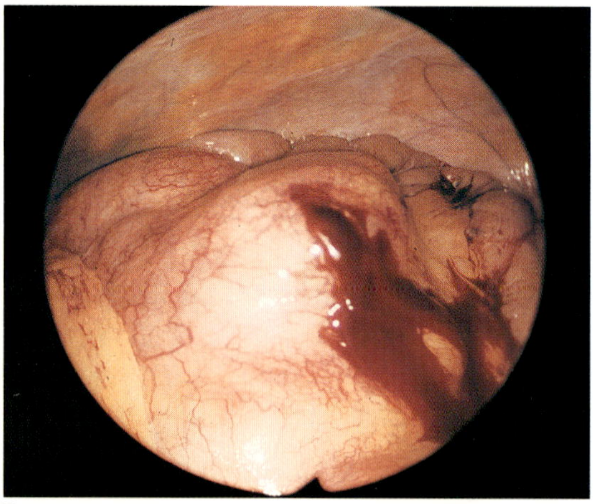

B

Case 3.9

A 62-year-old male with asymptomatic left upper quadrant (LUQ) mass. Past history of chronic lymphatic leukemia. CT scan confirmed a mass in the small bowel mesentery. Laparoscopic view of the LUQ with mass protruding and infiltrating a loop of jejunal mesentery. The palpating probe is on the mass. Dx: Histiocytic lymphoma.

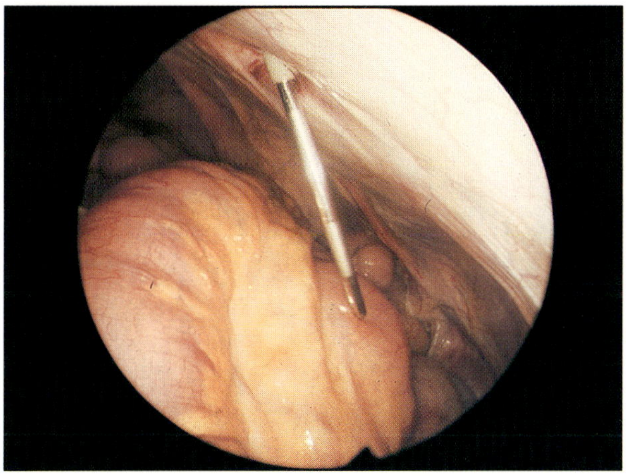

Case 3.10*A* and *B*

A 45-year-old female with weight loss and fever. The workup included a CT scan (Fig. 3.10**A**) that illustrates peripancreatic and periaortic nodal enlargement that surrounds a patent splenic vein. Figure 3.10**B** demonstrates lymphadenopathy originating from the lesser sac. The stomach is in the foreground, and the palpating probe is lifting the liver upwards. The thin lesser omentum is clearly visible. Dx: Non-Hodgkin's lymphoma.

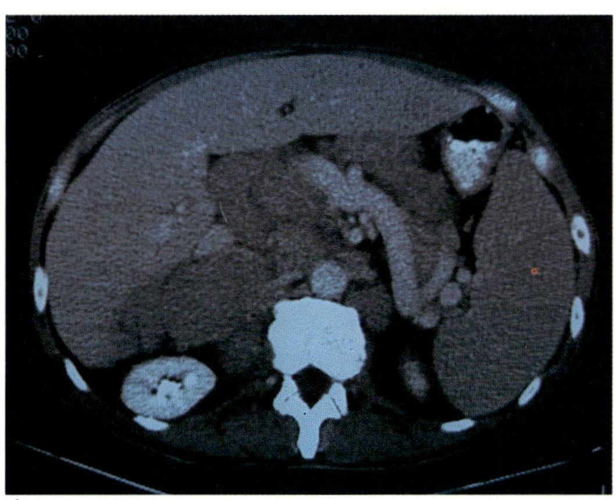

A

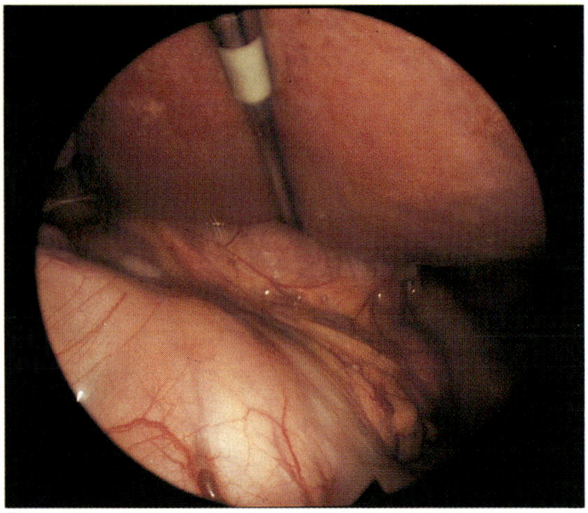

B

Case 3.11*A–C*

A 72-year-old female presented with fever, tender RLQ mass, and RLQ pain. The presumptive diagnosis was appendiceal abscess. No response to antibiotics prompted a CT scan (Fig. 3.11**A**), which shows a right lower retroperitoneal mass pushing the bladder upwards and to the left. Sonographic needle aspiration was nondiagnostic. Figure 3-11**B** demonstrates retroperitoneal lymphadenopathy pushing the bladder upwards. The patient is in steep Trendelenburg with the palpating probe depressing the sigmoid colon. Figure 3-11**C** shows biopsy site with lancet-shaped biopsy forceps. Dx: Non-Hodgkin's lymphoma.

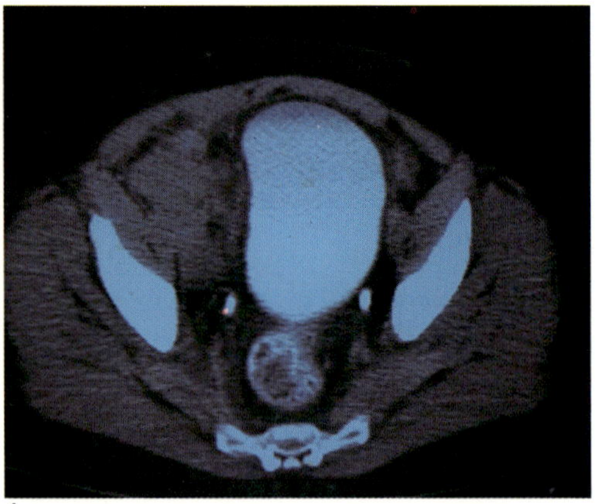

A

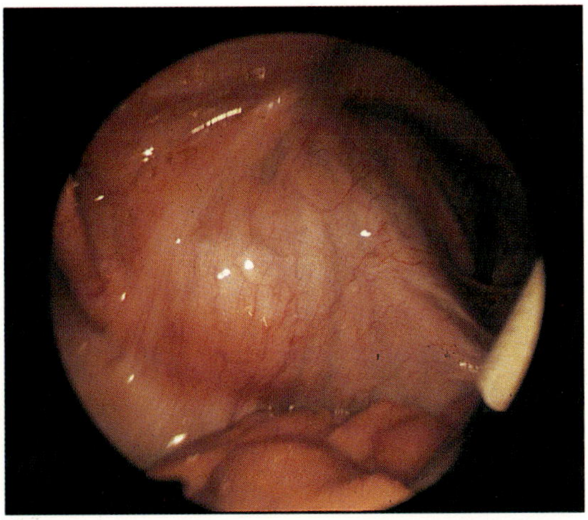

B

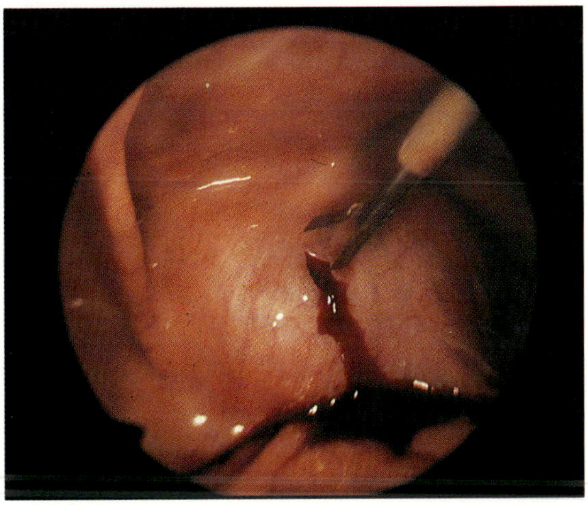

C

Case 3.12

A 56-year-old male with past history of Hodgkin's disease presented with fever and a pelvic mass on CT scan. Sonographic aspiration was nondiagnostic. Laparoscopic view of the pelvis with palpating probe elevating the sigmoid colon. Small bowel is in the foreground. Lymphadenopathy projects up from the pelvic retroperitoneum. Dx: Non-Hodgkin's lymphoma.

Cases 3.6 through 3.12 show examples of retroperitoneal lymphomatous disease that are approachable via the laparoscope. This modality is important in that if adequate tissue can be obtained with directed biopsies, formal laparotomy can be avoided. The procedure almost always

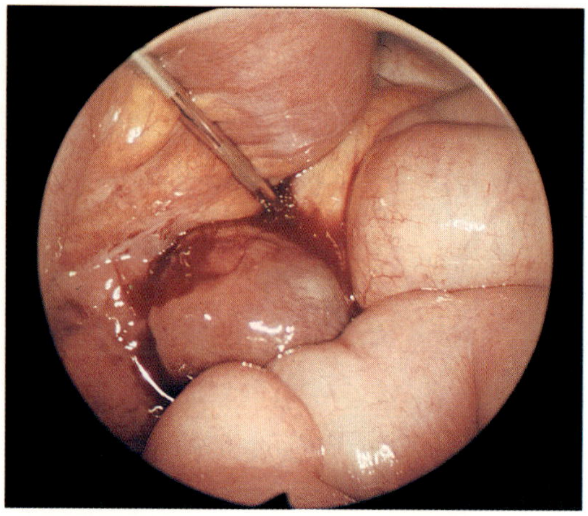

requires manipulation of viscera to visualize the retroperitoneal process. A second and even a third puncture site may be needed both to move viscera and to biopsy through. The use of a tilt table is also helpful to allow the bowel to "fall away" from the planned biopsy site. This mode of diagnosis should be considered when preoperative scans or radiographs demonstrate displacement of viscera or when the process is palpable. It is not appropriate in minimal retroperitoneal adenopathy. In the author's experience, this technique will yield a positive tissue diagnosis in approximately 85% of patients. If lymphomatous disease is suspected, a concomitant liver biopsy (or biopsies) is (are) indicated at the same time. Tissue samples for cell marker studies should also be obtained. In all of the patients presented above, no peripheral adenopathy was present, and all bone marrow examinations were negative. Skinny needle aspiration is usually unrewarding in the diagnosis of lymphomatous disease, as cytological diagnosis is not as definitive as it is in histological specimens. The added advantage of obtaining core samples is the ability to perform marker studies.

Case 3.13*A* and *B*

A 56-year-old male with fever and weight loss. CT scan (Fig. 3.13**A**) demonstrates bilateral iliac nodal enlargement. Significant bladder compression is seen on the right. Skinny needle aspiration was nondiagnostic. Laparoscopic view (Fig. 3.13**B**) showed upward displacement of the urinary bladder. Palpating probe is in the foreground depressing the sigmoid colon. Dx: Metastatic transitional cell carcinoma. Although not an example of lymphomatous disease, this case again demonstrates the ease of obtaining retroperitoneal biopsies when scanning demonstrates displacement of viscera. The primary was subsequently found in the urinary bladder after the laparoscopy.

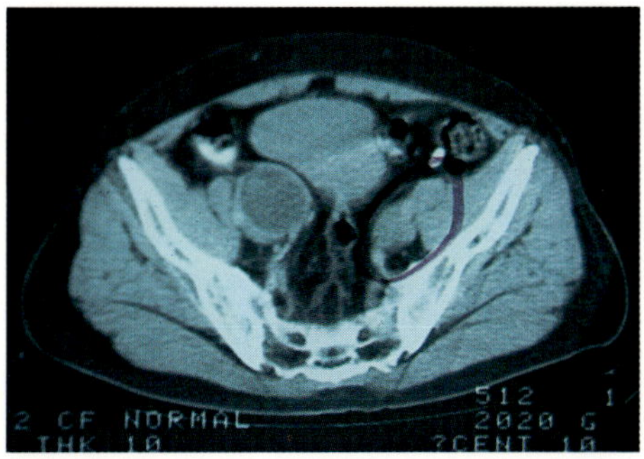

A

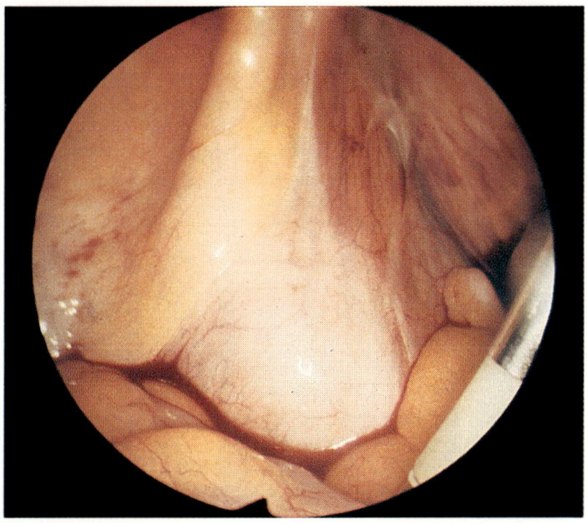

B

Case 3.14*A–C*

A 56-year-old male presented with weight loss, back pain, and epigastric fullness. CT scan showed a lesion in the body of the pancreas. Skinny needle aspiration was nondiagnostic. Laparoscopic view (Fig. 3.14**A**) of pancreatic mass pushing the left lobe of the liver superiorly. Stomach is in the foreground. Figure 3.14**B** shows grasping forceps entering from the left and scissors entering from the right. Lesser omentum placed on stretch to allow cutting of the avascular lesser omentum (Fig. 3.14**C**). Closeup view of the pancreatic biopsy. Dx: Adenocarcinoma of the pancreas. In the author's experience, skinny needle aspiration of the pancreas is the method of choice for obtaining a tissue diagnosis of pancreatic body lesion. However, occasionally, nondiagnostic samples will necessitate other means of making the diagnosis. There is no question that it is a lot simpler and easier for the patient if laparoscopy and directed biopsy are positive, rather than having to perform formal laparotomy. It is not accomplishable in every case. The first picture in this series demonstrates an important diagnostic point. The left lobe of the liver should lay on the anterior aspect of the stomach. If the liver is lifted off the stomach, then either something is in the lesser sac pushing it off (as in this case), or there is pathology in the undersurface of the left lobe of the liver. It is one of the reasons why the placement of a second puncture is necessary for a thorough examination of the abdominal cavity with the laparoscope.

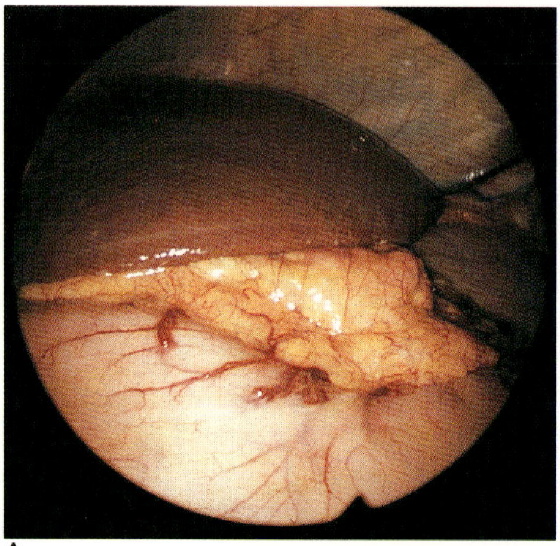

A

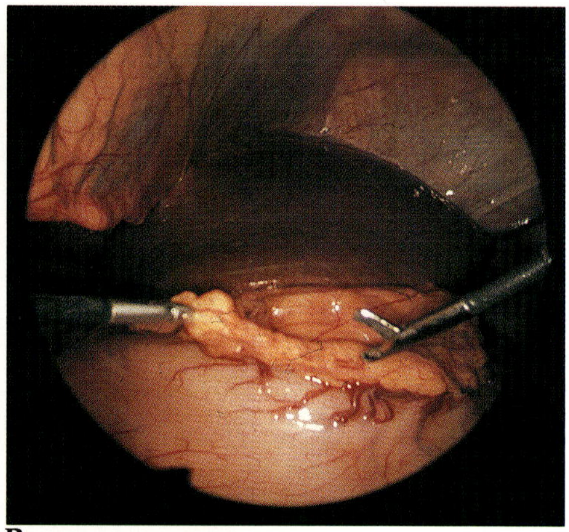

B

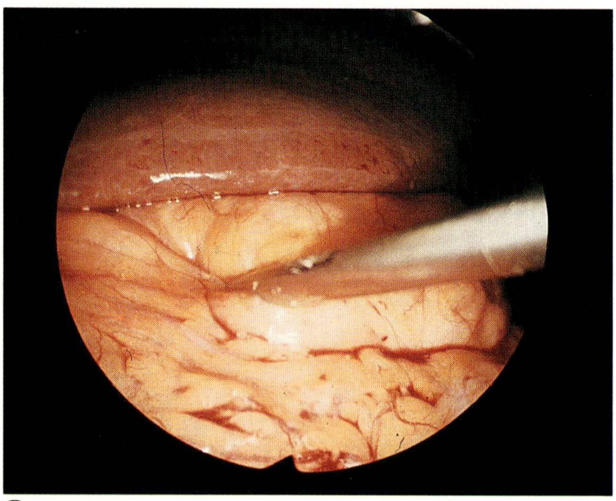

C

4

LIVER DISEASE

The laparoscope has been used in the evaluation of liver diseases for many years by hepatologists and gastroenterologists. Using it provides the advantage of visualization of approximately 80 to 85% of the liver surface. The laparoscopist can not examine the bare area or the posterior aspect of the right lobe. One also cannot visualize the interior of the liver unless there is a manifestation of the process on the surface, which in the author's experience is not uncommon. There are two primary indications for laparoscopy for the surgeon in the evaluation of focal liver defects as defined by either sonography, CT scan, or magnetic resonance imaging. The most common is the obtaining of tissue by means of directed biopsy under visual control to obtain a firm histological diagnosis. In patients who are potential candidates for hepatic resection, using the laparoscope is an excellent method of finding other disease that may preclude laparotomy, and thus spare the patient an unneeded exploration. The author has not used laparoscopy in the evaluation of chronic hepatic disorders and, therefore, that is beyond the scope of this text.

Many internists will opt for blind percutaneous liver biopsy as the first invasive procedure, depending on the location and number of defects. However, the diagnostic accuracy of blind percutaneous biopsy varies between 55 and 90%, as reported in the literature. CT scan-guided biopsy is more accurate than blind biopsy when large-bore biopsy needles are used, but large amounts of CT scan time may be necessary, which may not be practical in many hospital settings. Laparoscopic liver biopsy offers several advantages over each of the other biopsy techniques. In the author's experience, its diagnostic accuracy is 95%. It is common to find other significant pathology that was not discovered on the noninvasive scan. The risk of post-biopsy bleeding is slightly less with the laparoscopic approach. Approximately 20% of the author's patients have had a previous failed percutaneous biopsy. All of these were definitively diagnosed by laparoscopy.

The field of vision with laparoscopy is far superior to the operative field of vision with minilaparotomy. For that reason the author no longer performs open liver biopsy by means of the minilaparotomy route.

BENIGN DISEASE

Case 4.1

A 68-year-old female with known ovarian cacinoma demonstrated a left lobe liver defect on CT scan as part of a follow-up examination. The patient had received radiotherapy of the pelvis. Laparoscopic view of the upper abdomen demonstrated a large hemangioma on the lateral aspect of the lateral segment of the left lobe of the liver. The stomach and lesser omentum are on the *right,* and the round ligament can be seen in the *top left.* Biopsy of hepatic hemangioma is contraindicated. The diagnosis is established by visual means only. The clinical importance of this benign finding in the presence of known malignancy is obvious. Systemic chemotherapy was not needed.

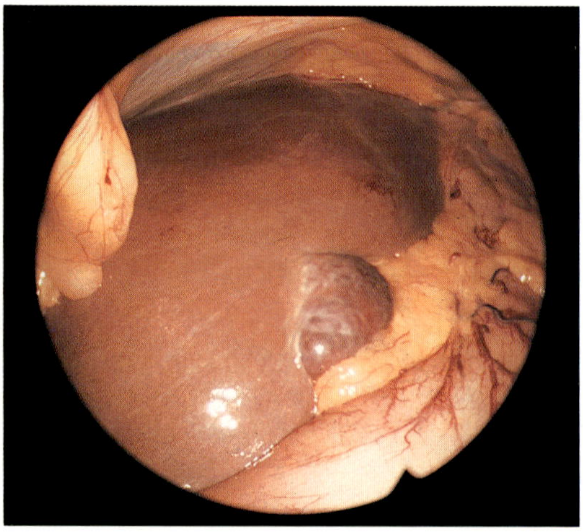

Case 4.2

A 65-year-old female presented with right upper quadrant (RUQ) pain. Sonogram demonstrated gallstones and a mass in the right lobe of the liver medial to the gallbladder. CT scan did not demonstrate a lesion. Laparoscopic view of undersurface of the right lobe of the liver is seen. Palpating probe is lifting liver superiorly, putting a flimsy adhesion on stretch. There is a 2-cm, firm, smooth tumor in the medial segment of the left lobe of the liver adjacent to the gallbladder and indenting it. The duodenum and hepatic flexure of the colon are in the foreground. Dx: Hepatic adenoma. Hepatic adenoma is the presumptive diagnosis, as biopsy is risky in these highly vascular tumors. The palpating probe is helpful in determining consistency of hepatic tumors. Adenomas are very firm and resist movement. Despite a strong recommendation for cholecystectomy and removal of the adenoma, the patient refused and has since been lost to follow-up.

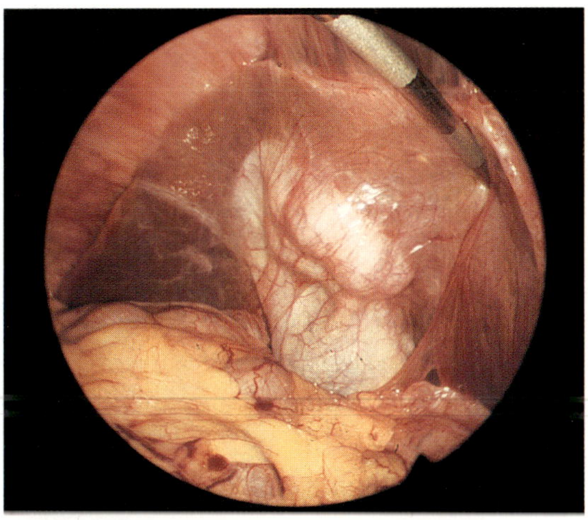

Case 4.3

A 42-year-old female presented with a fever of undetermined origin. The workup revealed a defect in the left lobe of the liver. The rest of the evaluation was negative, except for a markedly elevated sedimentation rate, high SGOT and SGPT, and increased WBC count. Laparoscopic view of the lateral segment of the left lobe of the liver showed extensive necrosis in various stages of progression. There is scar formation on the inferior edge, hemorrhagic areas in the central portion, and frank necrosis on the *left*. A small segment of the stomach is visible in the *foreground*. The falciform ligament is seen in the background. Dx: Hepatic necrosis etiology unknown. The preoperative diagnosis was thought to be meta-

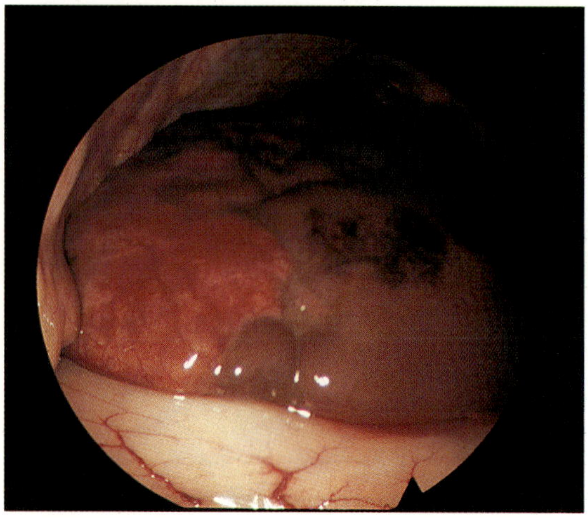

static disease. The surprise finding of necrosis eventually resolved spontaneously with normalization of all liver chemistries over a 6-month period. Etiology was never ascertained.

Case 4.4*A* and *B*

A 73-year-old male presented with weight loss. The evaluation included a CT scan that was read as most likely a tumor of the left lobe of the liver (Fig. 4.4**A**). A primary and metastatic workup was negative. Laparoscopic. view of lesion on undersurface of the lateral segment of the left lobe of the liver is seen (Fig. 4.4**B**). Its characteristics are unlike those of hemangioma, but are more like those of a primary liver tumor. The second puncture probe is seen lifting the lateral segment. The lesser omentum is

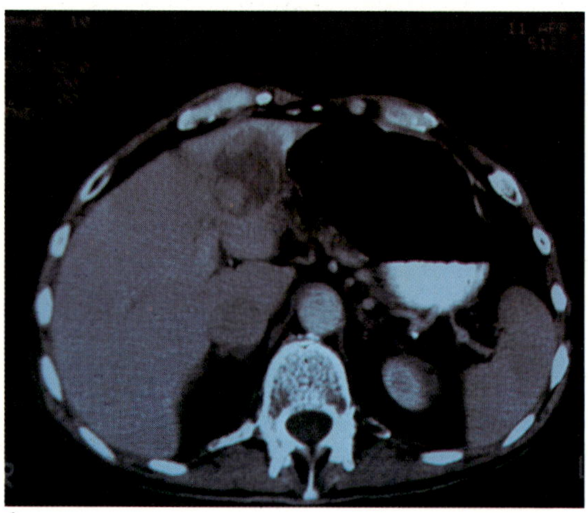

A

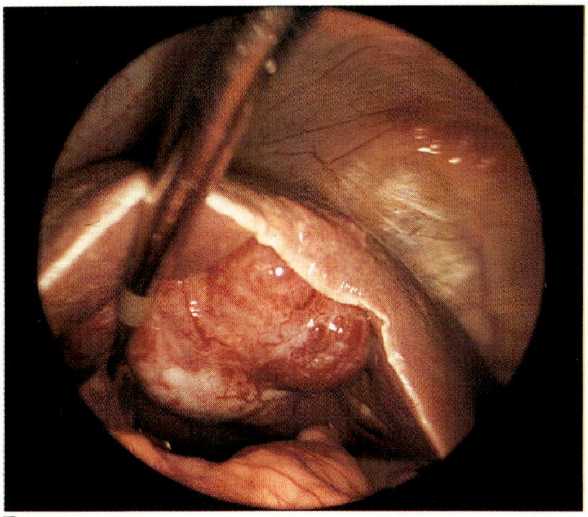

B

in the *foreground*, and the diaphragm is in the *background*. The author could not differentiate between a solid liver tumor or hemangioma at the time of laparoscopy. Therefore, a directed liver biopsy was not undertaken. It is important to rule out a hemangioma completely before biopsy is performed. In the majority of situations, this is straightforward, as hemangiomas have a typical spongy feel to them, which can be readily ascertained by placing the second puncture probe on them. In cases of sclerosed hemangiomas, ruling them out can be impossible. This patient underwent angiography, which was consistent with, but not diagnostic of, a primary hepatic tumor. Laparotomy and resection of the lateral segment revealed a sclerosed hemangioma.

Case 4.5*A* and *B*

A 65-year-old male 3 years status post-excision of a melanoma of the foot underwent routine surveillance with CT scan (Fig. 4.5**A**). A defect in the left lobe of the liver is seen. Two attempts at blind percutaneous biopsy were unsuccessful. Laparoscopic view of large partially sclerosed hemangioma originating from the medial segment of the left lobe of the liver is shown (Fig. 4.5**B**). This diaphragm is in the *background;* the round ligament is superior and to the *right;* and the tip of the gallbladder can be seen *just behind* the hemangioma. Dx: Partially sclerosed hemangioma. The purplish color of hemangiomata may be difficult to differentiate from that of melanoma. In this case, the importance was paramount. Therefore, a biopsy of the whitish sclerosed portion of the hemangioma was performed, the author knowing the potential risk of bleeding. The lancet-shaped biopsy forceps is ideal for taking superficial biopsies as was necessary in this case. It was indeed fortunate that the two blind attempts at biopsy failed.

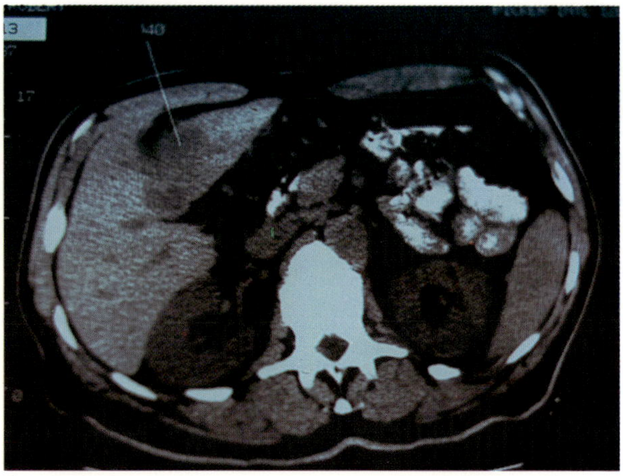

A

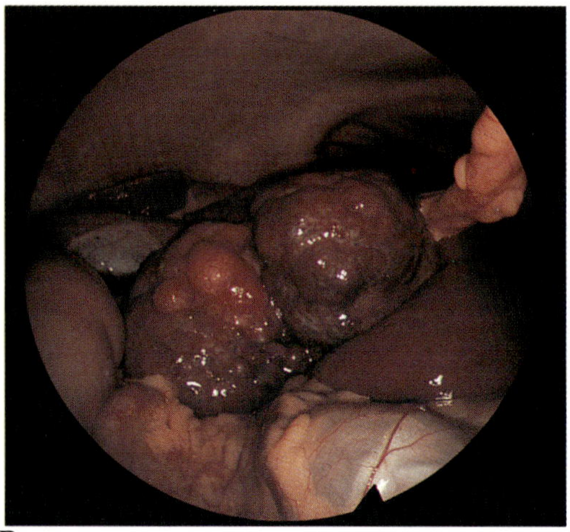

B

Case 4.6

A 66-year-old female 2 years post-abdominoperineal resection for adenocarcinoma of the rectum underwent CT scan as part of a follow-up examination. Two defects were found in the right lobe of the liver. The carcino embryonic antigen (CEA) was normal. Laparoscopic view of the right lobe and medial segment of the left lobe revealed a 2-cm benign cyst on the edge of the medial segment of the left lobe. The cyst was in the same location as demonstrated on the CT scan. The gallbladder has an omental adhesion draped over it, and the diaphragm is in the *background.* Although the preoperative CT scan was consistent with benign cysts, they were not present on a previous scan before the abdominoperineal resection. Therefore, laparoscopy was undertaken. Clear liver cysts can be aspirated laparoscopically but should only be performed if the cyst is symptomatic. The diagnosis is sufficient based on the visual appearance.

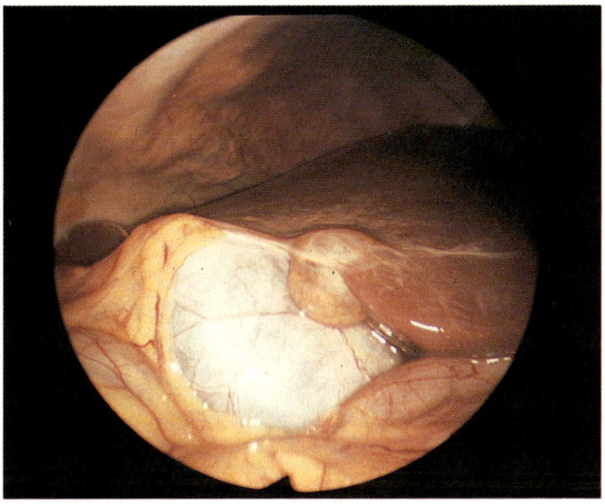

Case 4.7

A 42-year-old male presented with fever and weight loss. An extensive evaluation revealed abnormal liver chemistry, which prompted a CT scan of the abdomen. Diffuse infiltration of the liver was documented. A blind percutaneous biopsy was nondiagnostic. Laparoscopic view of the lateral segment of the left lobe of the liver shows extensive infiltration by whitish firm lesions. The stomach is in the *foreground,* and the diaphragm is in the *background.* Dx: Sarcoid of the liver. The preoperative differential diagnosis was between lymphoma and sarcoid. In general, the more infiltrative the process, the easier and more accurate the biopsy. This is clear from the view of the lateral segment. A biopsy anywhere in this part of the liver would have been diagnostic.

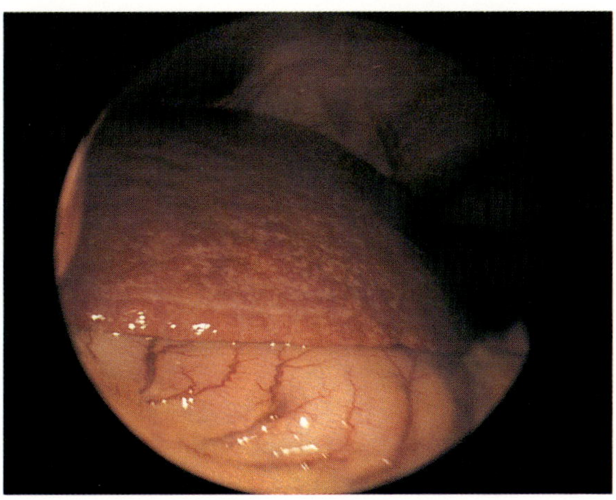

Case 4.8

A 75-year-old male underwent gastrointestinal evaluation for abdominal pain. While the barium contrast studies were negative, a sonogram revealed a mass in the left lobe of the liver. CT scan was consistent with a primary tumor, although a hemangioma could not be completely excluded. A nuclear scan was not consistent with hemangioma. Laparoscopic view of the lateral segment demonstrated a typical hemangioma. Notice the easy compressibility with the palpating probe. A very thickened capsule that is seen frequently with sclerosed hemangioma is visible just above the probe. The diaphragm is in the background. Nonsclerosed hemangiomata are usually easy to diagnose with noninvasive scanning techniques, especially magnetic resonant imaging. However, no test is 100% accurate when sclerosis occurs. In the author's opinion, laparoscopy is the best way of differentiating, short of open laparotomy. The insertion of a second puncture with palpating probe is mandatory.

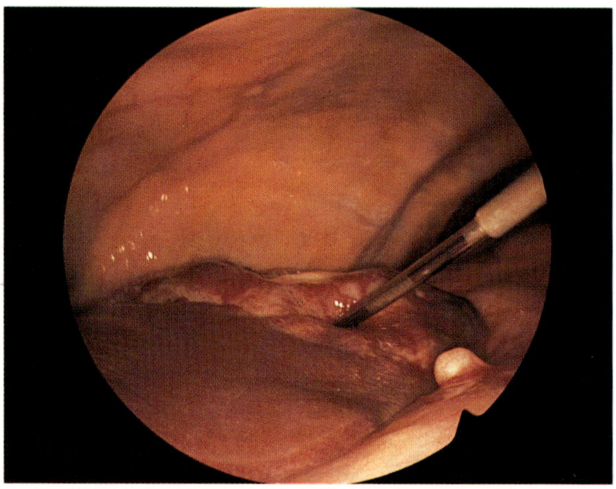

Case 4.9

A 48-year-old female presented with right upper quadrant abdominal pain. Sonography demonstrated gallstones and a mass in the medial aspect of the right lobe of the liver. CT scan confirmed the sonogram, and it was not consistent with a hemangioma. Laparoscopic view of the medial aspect of the right lobe demonstrated a subcapsular mass of slight yellowish-red color just above the palpating probe. It was firm to compression. The diaphragm is in the *background,* and a small portion of the falciform ligament is visible on the *far right.* Dx: Focal nodular hyperplasia. Focal nodular hyperplasia is a benign epithelial tumor of the liver. It is usually asyptomatic and must be differentiated from other tumors of the liver. Resectional therapy is reserved for those that obtain size sufficient to produce symptoms.

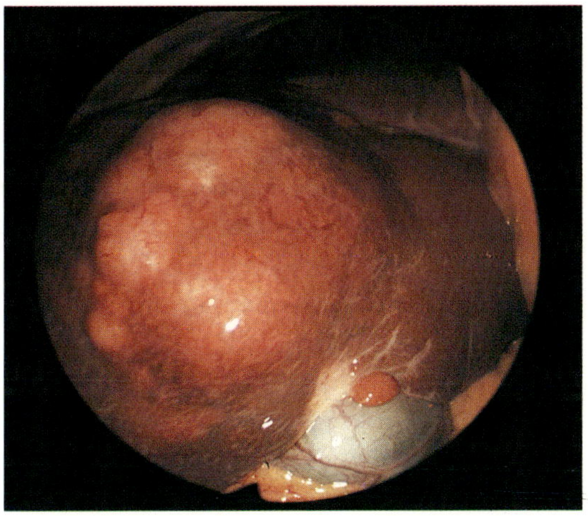

Case 4.10

A 74-year-old female 5 years status post-mastectomy for carcinoma developed an elevated alkaline phosphatase on routine screening that led to a CT scan that demonstrated a defect in the lateral segment of the left lobe of the liver. Premastectomy scans were normal. Laparoscopic view of the lateral segment of the left lobe with a typical hemangioma on its anterior surface is shown. Notice the bluish discoloration around the

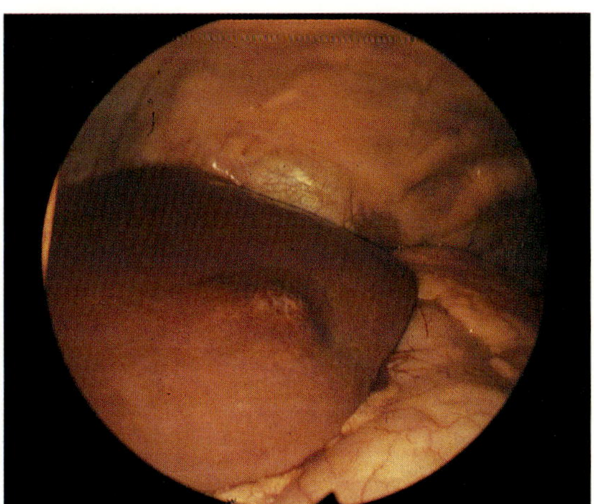

lesion. The hemangioma was compressible with the secondary palpating probe. The diaphragm is in the *background,* and the stomach is underneath the lateral segment. The preoperative diagnosis was metastatic breast carcinoma. The findings in this case underline the necessity of pursuing a tissue diagnosis in almost all cases of metastatic cancer, as proper treatment is dependent on correct assessment. In this case, there was no metastatic disease. This patient is without evidence of disease 5 years later.

Case 4.11

A 40-year-old male with known cerebral lymphoma treated by means of radiotherapy presented with abnormal liver function tests. Workup for systemic lymphoma was negative. There was a past history of alcohol abuse. CT scan demonstrated several filling defects in both lobes of the liver. Laparoscopic view of the lateral segment of the left lobe of the liver showing distorted surface architecture consistent with cirrhosis. There is no suggestion of lymphoma. The diaphragm is in the *background,* and the parietal peritoneum does not demonstrate any dilated veins that would be compatible with portal hypertension. Dx: Schistosomiasis. Liver defects can be caused by regenerative nodules in cirrhosis. There was no evidence of lymphoma grossly or microscopically. The surprise finding of schistosomiasis on the liver biopsy may be the etiology of the cirrhotic pattern. Schistosomatic liver involvement usually produces a presinusoidal portal hypertension, although there was no evidence of hypertension in this patient at laparoscopy. Appropriate antimicrobial therapy was instituted.

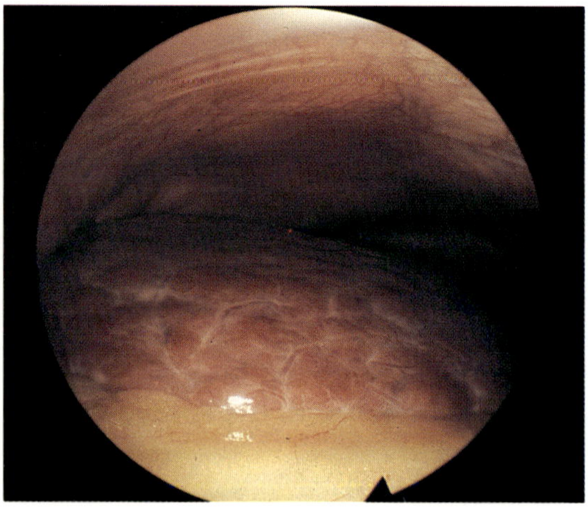

Case 4.12

A 47-year-old female 4 years status post-left mastectomy presented with upper abdominal pain. As part of her workup a CT scan was performed that demonstrated two defects in the liver, one in each lobe. A premastectomy liver scan had not been done. The lesion in the right lobe was consistent with a benign liver cyst. However, the defect in the left lobe was thought to be a metastatic deposit. Laparoscopic view of the undersurface of the lateral segment of the left lobe demonstrated a typical benign cyst. The palpating probe is elevating the segment. The lesser omentum is clearly seen below the liver with a small portion of the stomach visible on the *far right.* The diaphragm with its phrenic vessels is seen in the background. Dx: Benign liver cyst. There are several important points in this case. Firstly, the etiology of the defects was clarified by means of laparoscopy. The findings were somewhat at odds with the preprocedure CT scan. Secondly, the importance of a second puncture is evident, in that the only way this cyst would have been seen is by lifting the lateral segment. There was no anterior surface manifestation. Lastly, the biopsy of a cyst of the liver is contraindicated if it contains bile. Clear cysts, like those seen here, can be safely aspirated, but only if they are symptomatic.

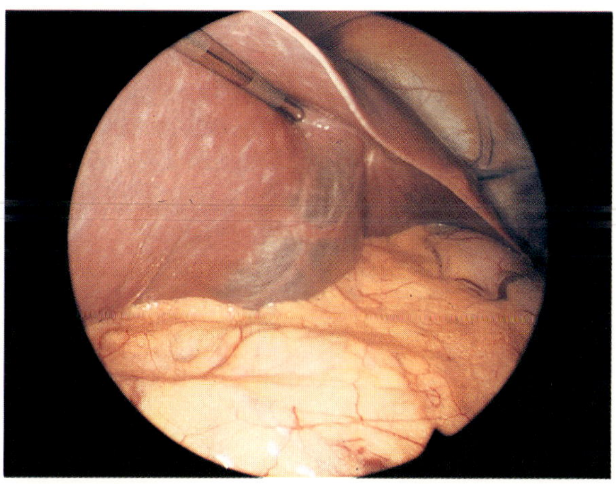

Case 4.13

A 70-year-old male presented with obstructive jaundice. A workup revealed an ampullary carcinoma. A CT scan showed dilated intrahepatic ducts and several defects in both lobes of the liver. A blind percutaneous liver biopsy was negative for metastatic disease. Laparoscopic view of the medial segment of the left lobe is shown. The palpating probe is in

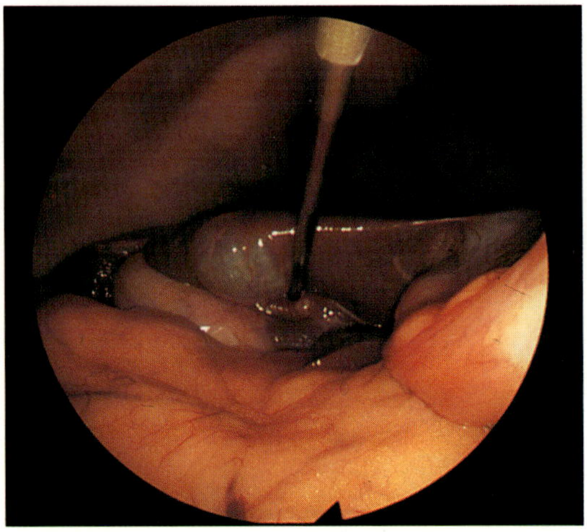

the middle of two lesions. The upper one is a typical benign clear cyst. The tip of the probe is on a small lesion that was not appreciated on the CT scan or sonogram. The gallbladder is visible to the left of the cyst and is tense on palpation. There were multiple other cystic structures in the right lobe as well. The round ligament is on the *far right,* and the omentum is in the foreground. Dx: Multiple benign liver cysts. This patient was considered nonoperable based on the preoperative CT scan. As tissue proof of metastatic disease was not present, laparoscopy was performed. As a direct result of the laparoscopic findings, the patient underwent a potentially curable Whipple procedure. In the author's experience, the laparoscope is an ideal tool in the evaluation of metastatic liver disease. There will be both upgrading and downgrading in terms of operability. But most importantly, the patient will benefit from the right procedure recommendation.

Case 4.14

A 68-year-old male presented with upper abdominal pain and a palpable mass in the epigastrium. The patient had a past history of toxoplasmosis. A CT scan showed a prominent left lobe and several focal defects. There was a small amount of ascitic fluid present. The liver function tests were normal. Laparoscopic view of the lateral segment of the left lobe demonstrated an exudate covering the liver. There are several small regenerative nodules clearly visible. The round ligament does not demonstrate portal hypertension. The omentum seen in the foreground is also exudate-covered. A small portion of the medial segment is seen at the *far left*. Dx: Cirrhosis. A nonbacterial exudative process secondary to cirrhosis is an occasional finding laparoscopically. It should not be confused with bacterial peritonitis. There was no clinical suspicion of cirrhosis before the laparoscopy. This surprise finding was confirmed by a directed biopsy. The etiology was never ascertained. Filling defects in cirrhosis are probably secondary to regenerating nodules and can be confused with malignant disease. The laparoscope is a good method for differentiating this.

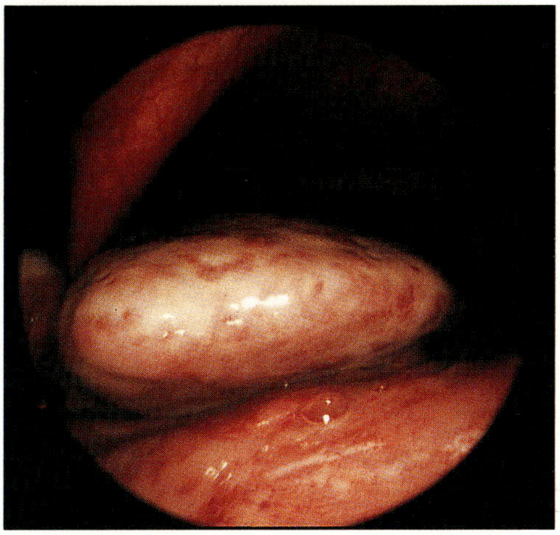

Case 4.15*A–C*

A 79-year-old female presented with an asymptomatic mass in the RUQ. CT scan showed a mass in the lateral portion of the right lobe of the liver consistent with either primary or metastatic disease (Fig. 4.15**A**). A thorough workup was negative. Laparoscopic view of the lateral aspect of the right lobe showed a mass under the surface with dilated vascular lakes prominent on the surface (Fig. 4.15**B**). The hepatic flexure of the

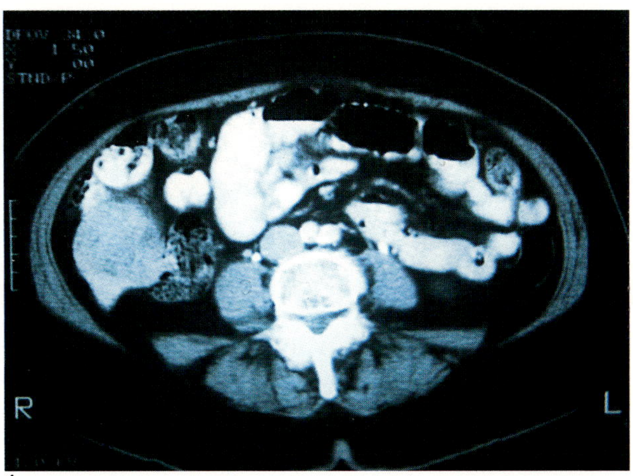

A

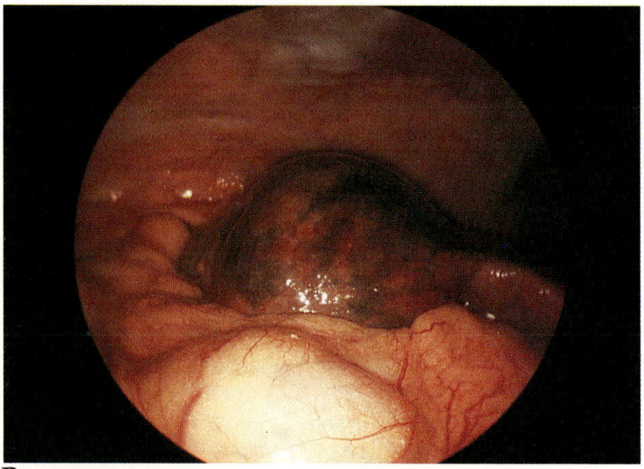

B

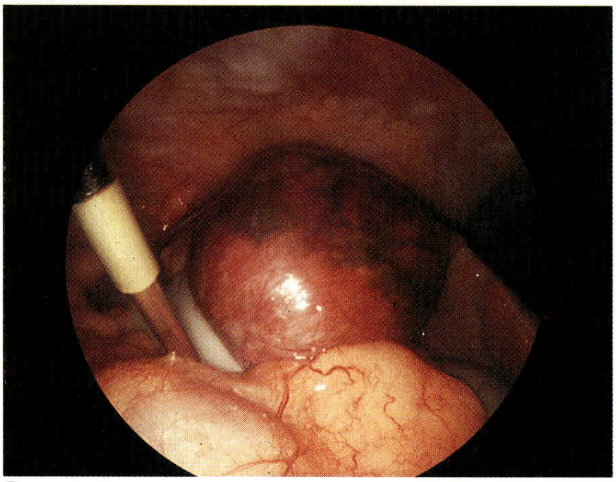

C

colon is seen in the foreground of the first picture. Figure 4.15**C** shows the second puncture probe lifting up the right lobe. A thick, whitish capsule is clearly visible now. The gallbladder is more medial and is not seen in the picture. It was normal. Dx: Ecchinococcal cyst. Ecchinococcal liver disease must be recognized by the examiner, as biopsy is contraindicated. The thick, whitish capsule is typical and should alert the viewer to the diagnosis. This case also points out the need for a second puncture probe. The first picture was the in situ view, and it is misleading as to the etiology of the mass. Post-procedure, a Casoni skin test was positive. Because of her age and associated medical problems, surgery was not recommended.

MALIGNANT DISEASE

Case 4.16*A–C*

A 54-year-old female presented with weight loss and increasing abdominal girth. The workup included a CT scan that showed a large defect in the right lobe of the liver (Fig. 4.16**A**). Percutaneous blind biopsy was nondiagnostic. Post-biopsy, the patient's hemoglobulin dropped significantly and developed abdominal and flank ecchymosis (Fig. 4.16**B**). Laparoscopic view of the right lobe showed an intact capsule that is tightly stretched over a mass in the right lobe (Fig. 4.16**C**). In the background an old blood clot can be seen attached to the abdominal wall. There is also a small amount of ascitic fluid present. The right transverse colon is just visible in the foreground and is displaced by the mass. Dx:

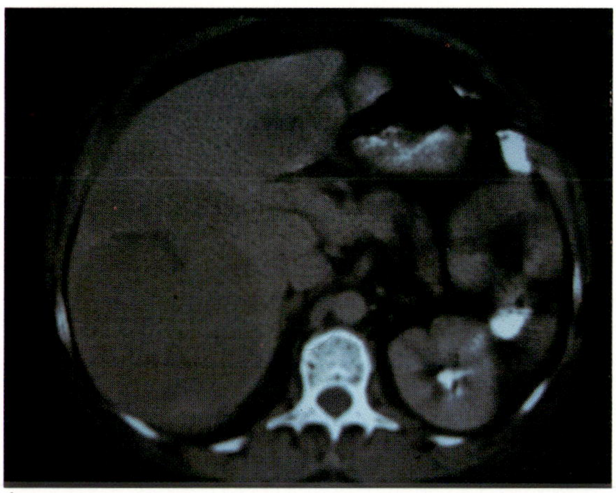

A

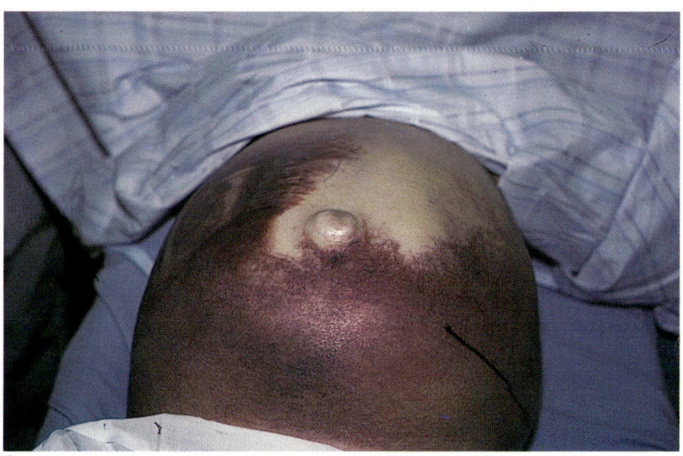

B

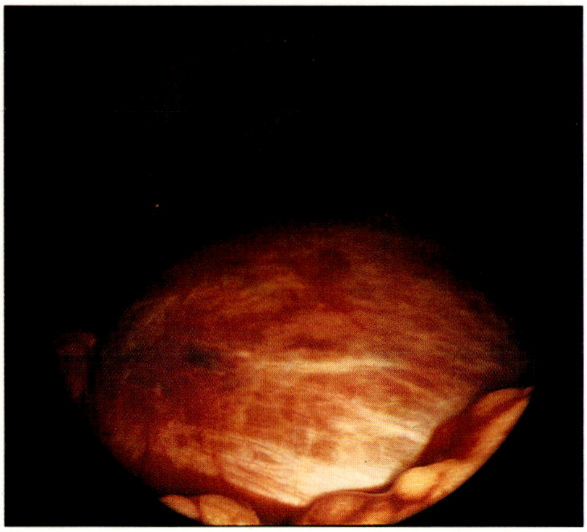

C

Undifferentiated carcinoma, primary unknown. Blind percutaneous biopsy is usually positive when the local lesion in the liver is of this size. The amount of post-biopsy bleeding was significant, as can be seen here. Even though the capsule of the liver was not directly invaded by tumor, the proper site to obtain tissue for biopsy is obvious. The surgeon should expect close to 100% tissue proof when the lesion attains this size.

Case 4.17*A–C*

A 68-year-old male presented with weight loss. CT scan performed as part of the workup revealed a mass in the body of the pancreas and metastatic liver disease (Fig. 4.17**A**). A percutaneous blind liver biopsy was negative for tumor. Skinny needle aspiration of the pancreatic mass was nondiagnostic. Laparoscopic view of the lateral segement of the left lobe demonstrated two metastatic lesions next to the falciform ligament (Fig. 4.17**B**). The diaphragm is in the background. Directed core biopsy showed carcinoma consistent with neuroendocrine primary. Figure 4.17**C** demonstrates the greater curvature of the stomach with a markedly dilated gastroepiploic vein consistent with segmental portal hypertension. The second puncture sleeve is positioned over the antrum of the stomach. On further review of the biopsy specimen, this tumor was classified as a nonsecreting islet cell adenocarconima. Skinny-needle aspiration was nondiagnostic in this patient. After multiple consultations, the patient decided not to be treated with chemotherapy. He has remained relatively asymptomatic over the last 2 years.

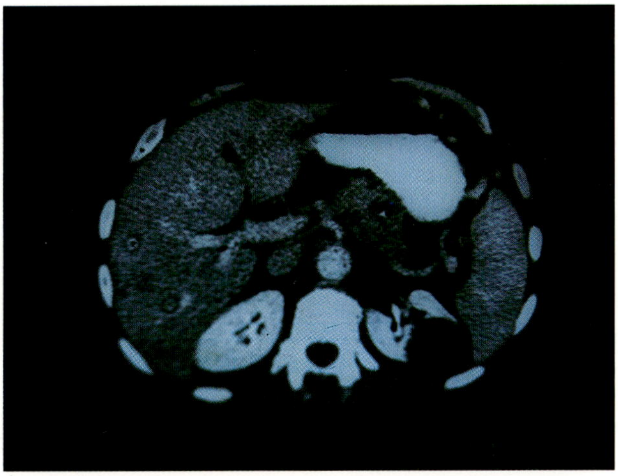

A

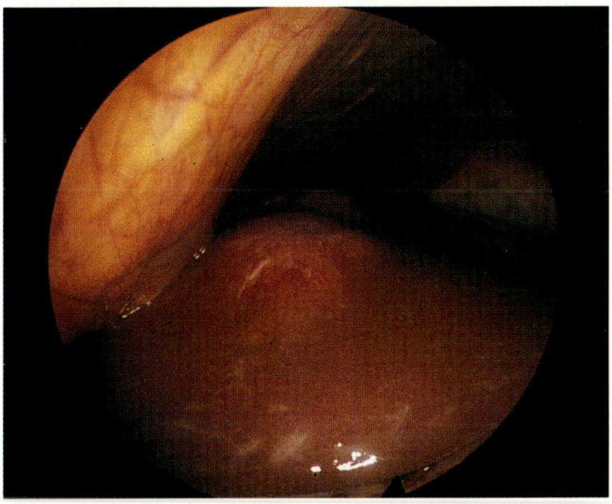

B

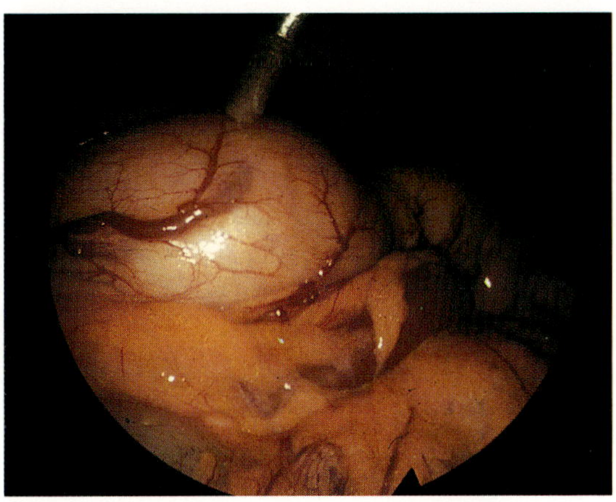

C

Case 4.18*A* and *B*

A 55-year-old female 10 years status post-left mastectomy for carcinoma presented with weight loss. CT scan was performed after liver function tests and showed elevation of the alkaline phosphatase. Figure 4.18**A** shows multiple defects in both lobes of the liver. Percutaneous blind liver biopsy was not diagnostic. Laparoscopic view of an enlarged lateral segment of the left lobe with multiple metastatic deposits (Fig. 4.18**B**). The round and falciform ligaments are on the *left,* and the diaphragm is in the *background.* A small portion of the stomach is visible in the foreground. Dx: Metastatic adenocarcinoma consistent with breast primary. The development of metastatic breast disease many years after mastectomy is unfortunately not uncommon. Its early detection is important as chemotherapeutic drugs are available for this disease. It is possible to obtain enough tissue for estrogen and progesterone receptors with laparoscopic biopsy forceps. This can be helpful in treatment options and prognosis predictions.

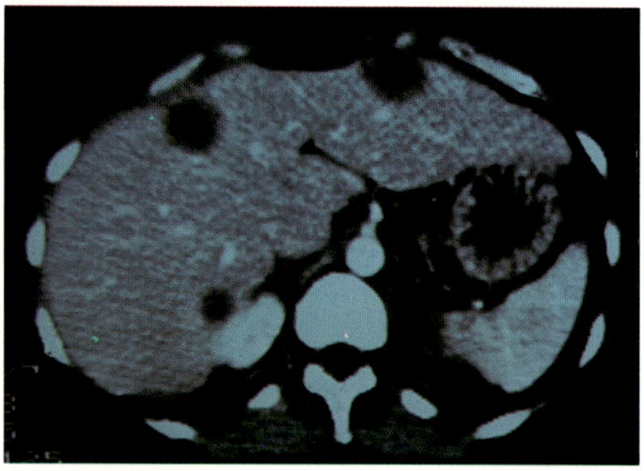

A

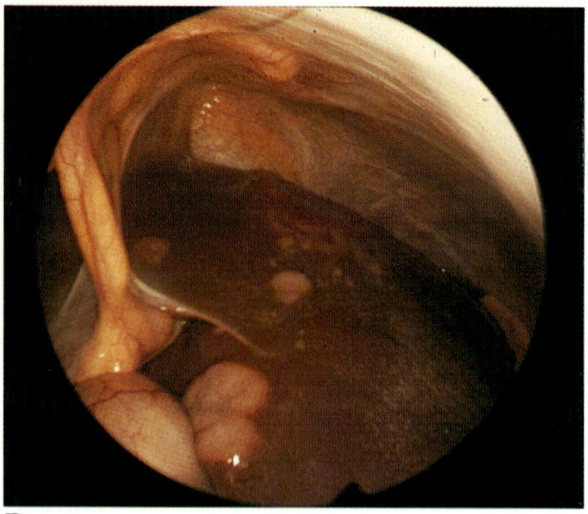

B

Case 4.19

A 68-year-old man presented with an elevated CEA 8 months status post-colon resection for adenocarcinoma. This prompted a workup that was negative, except for a CT scan that showed a hemangioma of the right lobe of the liver. Laparoscopic view of the edge of the lateral segment of the left lobe demonstrated a small metastatic deposit. The palpating probe is lifting the lateral segment off of the lessor omentum in the foreground. The falciform ligament is visible in the background. Dx: Metastatic adenocarcinoma consistent with colon primary. Laparoscopy was performed to clarify the liver pathology and to look for any evidence of metastatic disease to explain the elevation in CEA. There was a hemangioma in the right lobe, as predicted by the CT scan. However, the small metastatic lesion on the lateral segment was not detected on the CT scan or sonogram. This patient underwent angiography and then laparotomy based on the laparoscopic findings. No other metastatic disease was found, and the patient had an uneventful wedge resection of the lesion. The CEA returned to normal. In the author's experience, the laparoscope has been a helpful adjunct in the evaluation of metastatic disease to the liver. The laparoscope is a more sensitive technique for surface pathology, while the CT scan is more useful for deep pathology. The CT scan will not pick up lesions smaller than 1.5 cm, which gives the laparoscope an advantage for smaller surface lesions, as demonstrated clearly in this patient.

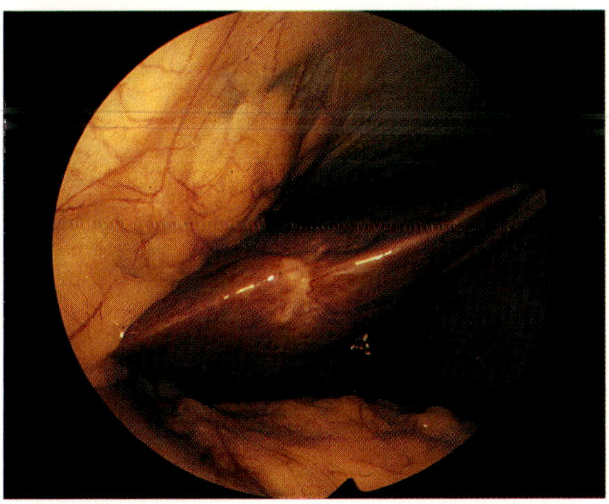

Case 4.20

A 66-year-old male 1 year status post-colon resection developed an elevated CEA. The workup was negative, including endoscopy and CT scan. The original lesion was a Duke's B1. Laparoscopic view of the lateral segment of the left lobe demonstrated a single metastatic lesion. The stomach is in the foreground, and the round ligament is in the center. A typical metastatic lesion is seen underneath the round ligament. Dx: Metastatic adenocarcinoma consistent with colon primary. This is another example of the benefit of laparoscopy. This peripherally located lesion was not detected by CT scan. The identification by laparoscopy is easy when the lesions are located on the surface. In fact, the more peripheral the lesion, the more likely detection is possible with the laparoscope. This patient had angiography and then left hepatic lobectomy. He developed disseminated disease 2 years later and died.

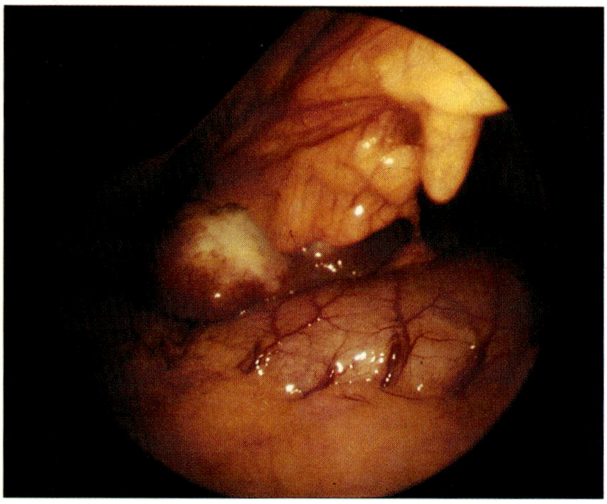

Case 4.21

A 72-year-old male presented with vague upper abdominal pain. The workup included a sonogram and CT scan that showed a mass in the pancreas and defects in both lobes of the liver. Skinny needle aspiration under sonographic guidance was nondiagnostic. Laparoscopic view of the left lobe of the liver revealed multiple small peripheral metastatic deposits and peritoneal seedings on the falciform ligament. The stomach is in the foreground. Dx: Adenocarcinoma consistent with biliary tract origin. This picture demonstrates several important laparoscopic principles. The lateral segment of the left lobe should be lying on the stomach wall. Any elevation of the liver off the stomach is abnormal, and a reason must be identified. The cause in this case is a large metastatic deposit within the confines of the lateral segment. Of course, the other causes usually emanate from the lessor sac or the stomach itself. It is also not uncommon to obtain other information besides the primary indication for performing the laparoscopy. In this case, peritoneal seeding was clearly identified.

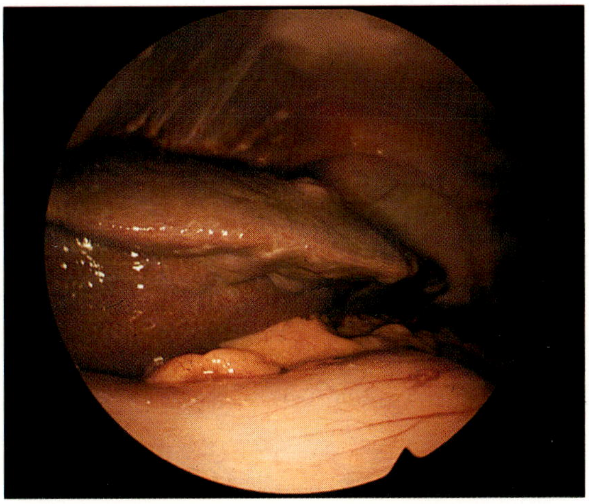

Case 4.22

A 52-year-old female presented with obstructive jaundice. Sonography showed dilated intrahepatic ducts and gallstones in a thickened gallbladder. Transhepatic cholangiography (THC) was read as being consistent with sclerosing cholangitis. A CT scan revealed a mass in the gallbladder fossa. Laparoscopic view of the liver and gallbladder demonstrated a cholestatic liver with several whitish metastatic deposits of the edge of the medial segment of the left lobe. The gallbladder-liver fossa junction is infiltrated by tumor. The gallbladder itself is firm and pale. Dx: Adenocarcinoma consistent with biliary tract origin. Laparoscopy was undertaken in an effort to clarify the discrepancies in the workup. Sclerosing cholangitis and metastatic liver disease can be difficult to separate on THC. The sonogram and CT scan were also

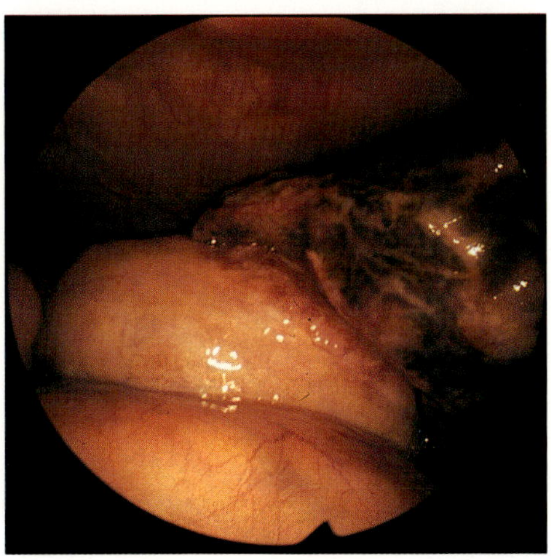

somewhat at odds with each other. In the author's opinion, laparoscopy is the procedure of choice in the diagnosis of carcinoma of the gallbladder. As the gallbladder can be seen in its entirety, the laparoscope is ideal in obtaining tissue proof of malignant disease. As metastatic disease is a common finding in gallbladder carcinoma, the biopsy can be obtained rather easily. There is usually no surgical treatment needed, except in the earliest of cases.

Case 4.23*A* and *B*

A 62-year-old female presented with weight loss and constipation. All results of the workup were negative, except for a CT scan that showed defects in both lobes of the liver, but more prominent on the left (Fig. 4.23**A**). Blind percutaneous biopsy was non-diagnostic. Laparoscopic view of the lateral segment of the left lobe showed a metastatic lesion with central umbilication that is typical of a gastrointestinal primary

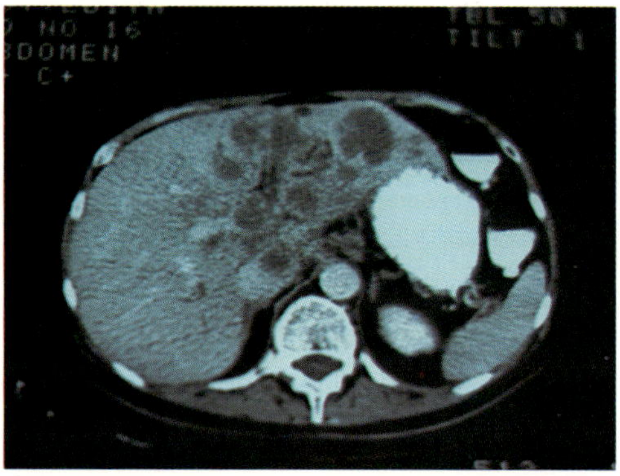

A

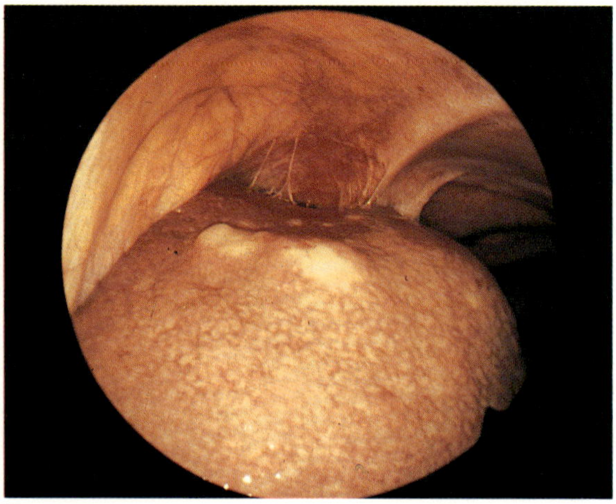

B

(Fig. 4.23**B**). The marked steatosis is an incidental finding. The falciform ligament is on the *left,* and the diaphragm is in the *background.* Dx: Mucin-producing adenocarcinoma. In the author's experience, there have not been any negative biopsies in focal liver pathology when the lesion can be visualized laparoscopically. In a small number of patients with previous surgery, adhesion formation will prevent direct visual biopsy. Most hepatologists will avoid left lobe biopsies, as the stomach wall is in close proximity. The left lobe is ideal for the laparoscope.

Case 4.24

A 60-year-old oriental male 18 months status post-Bilroth I gastrectomy for ulcer disease presented with upper abdominal pain and a palpable epigastric mass. Sonogram demonstrated a mass in the left lobe of the liver. Liver scan confirmed a defect (before CT scanning). A sudden increase in pain prompted laparoscopy. This is a view of the lateral segment of the liver nearly totally replaced by tumor. Notice the fresh blood on the parietal peritoneum. There is extensive adhesion formation to the undersurface of the lateral segment from the previous surgery. Dx: Hepatoma with spontaneous hemorrhage. Laparoscopy documented involvement of both lobes, which precluded a surgical approach to this very difficult clinical problem. This patient bled massively and died.

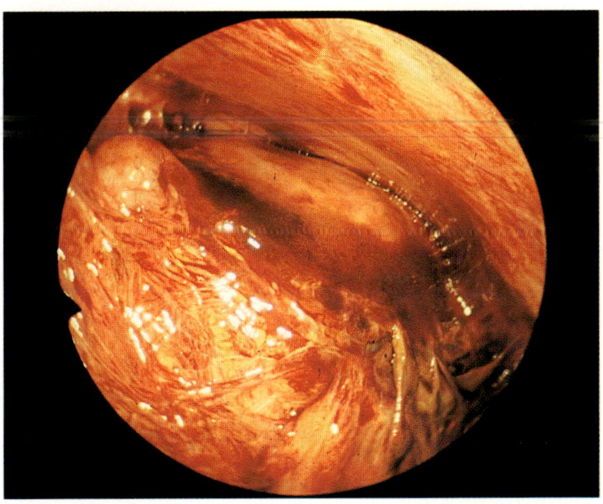

Case 4.25

A 76-year-old female 2 years status post-ileocolic resection for a leiomyosarcoma presented with weight loss. A workup was negative, except for a defect in the right lobe of the liver. Laparoscopic view of the lateral segment of the left lobe revealed a raised, firm lesion high on the lateral segment. Visualization of the right lobe was not possible because of extensive adhesion formation. The diaphragm is in the *background,* and the falciform ligament is on the *left.* Dx: Metastatic leiomyosarcoma. This patient was being evaluated for potential resection. The presence of a lesion in the right lobe was clear from the CT scan; however, the small lesion in the left lobe was not suspected based on the preprocedure evaluation. Even though the right side was not seen laparoscopically, important information was gained. Angiography and laparotomy were then avoided.

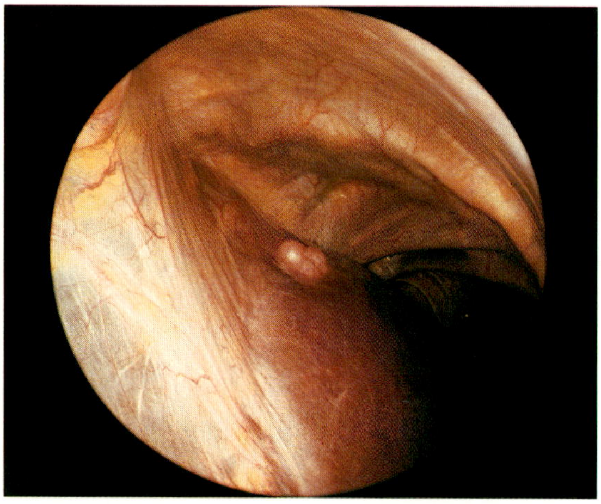

Case 4.26

An 84-year-old female presented with mild RUQ discomfort and an elevated alkaline phosphatase. A CT scan demonstrated a defect in the right lobe of the liver. Laparoscopic view of the right lobe demonstrated a highly vascular tumor with dilated vascular lakes on the surface. The "normal" liver is cirrhotic. The diaphragm is at the *top.* Dx: Hepatoma. Hepatomas are known to be highly vascular and are associated with an increased risk of post-biopsy hemorrhage. Laparoscopy has an advantage in that relatively avascular areas can be seen, and a biopsy can be performed on them directly. The presence of cirrhosis was unknown before laparoscopy but eliminates this patient as a candidate for resection.

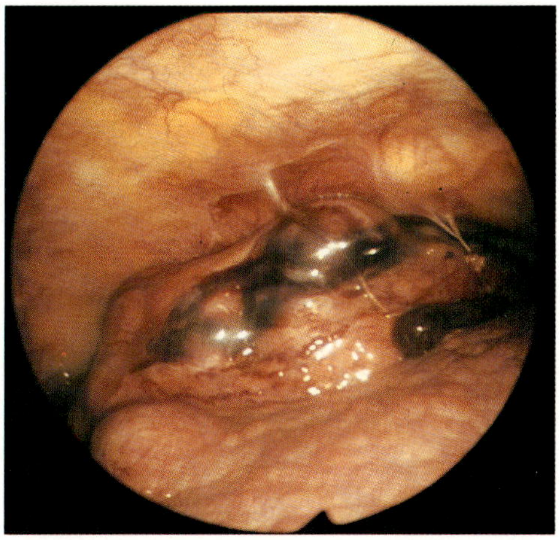

Case 4.27

A 35-year-old female with known chronic myelogenous leukemia presented with acute right lower quadrant pain while neutropenic from chemotherapy. A laparoscopy was performed to clarify the abdominal pain, and acute appendicitis was identified. An incidental finding of infiltration of the liver was seen. Three whitish masses are demonstrated in the medial segment of the left lobe. A normal gallbladder is visualized. Dx: Leukemic infiltration of the liver. In this patient, the laparoscopy was initiated because of an unclear clinical story in a complicated medical situation. Besides defining the etiology of the abdominal pain, information was obtained about the patient's primary disease as well. Appendectomy was uneventful.

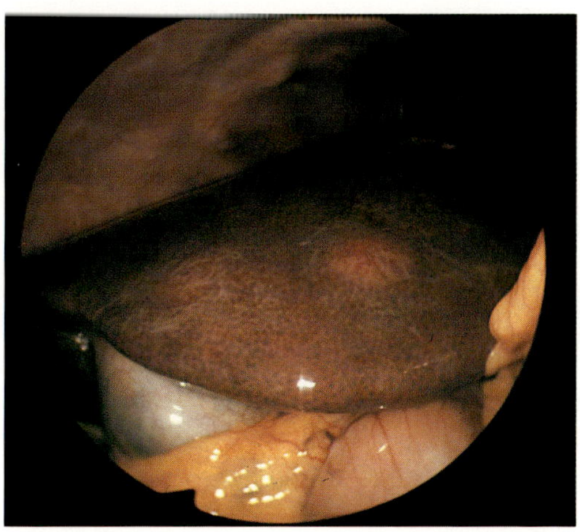

Case 4.28

A 62-year-old female with known myeloid metaplasia developed upper abdominal pain. A liver-spleen scan demonstrated defects in the spleen and the liver. The patient had had a left hemicolectomy for carcinoma 5 months before without any noticed splenic or liver pathology. Laparoscopic view of the spleen and the lateral segment of the left lobe demonstrated splenomegaly. There is a small subcapsular hematoma on the anterior edge of the spleen. The liver is enlarged but without gross defects. The diaphragm is in the *background,* and indentation from a rib is seen on the *right.* Dx: Myeloid metaplasia, splenomegaly with subcapsular hematoma. Laparoscopy was performed on this patient early in the author's experience before CT scanning was available. It is likely that a patient like this would not now be a candidate. It does demonstrate some salient points. The spleen can not ordinarily be seen during laparoscopy unless it is enlarged. The examiner should always percuss and palpate the LUQ before insertion of the laparoscope to avoid injury to any structure that should not be there. Indentations from the ribs are usually seen and are normal. The bluish discoloration on the edge of the liver is seen commonly in congested livers.

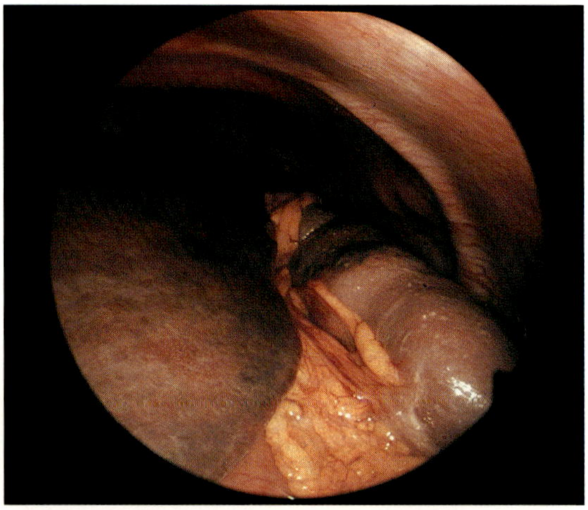

Case 4.29

A 78-year-old male with known multiple myeloma status post-excision of a melanoma of the leg presented with fullness in the epigastrium and decreased patient appetite. Liver scan showed several defects in the right lobe of the liver. Percutaneous blind biopsy was nondiagnostic. Laparoscopic view of the right lobe of the liver with a large subcapsular mass can be clearly seen above the gallbladder. There is a slight bluish discoloration lateral to the gallbladder. The diaphragm is in the *background*. Dx: Melanoma. The differential of the metaastatic disease was important here in that a different chemotherapeutic regimen would be needed, depending on the histology of the liver lesions. Even though the process was subcapsular, directed biopsy was straightforward.

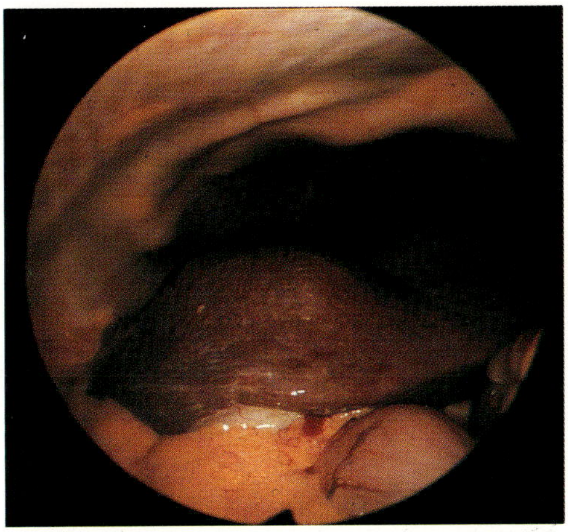

Case 4.30

A 68-year-old female presented 1 year status post-anterior resection for carcinoma with an elevated CEA. CT scan showed a peripherally placed metastatic lesion in the right lobe of the liver. Laparoscopic view of the lateral segment of the left lobe demonstrated several 1-cm or less lesions near the edge of the lateral segment. The diaphragm is in the *background* with the left phrenic vessels seen. The stomach is beneath the lateral segment. Dx: Metastatic colon carcinoma. This is another demonstration

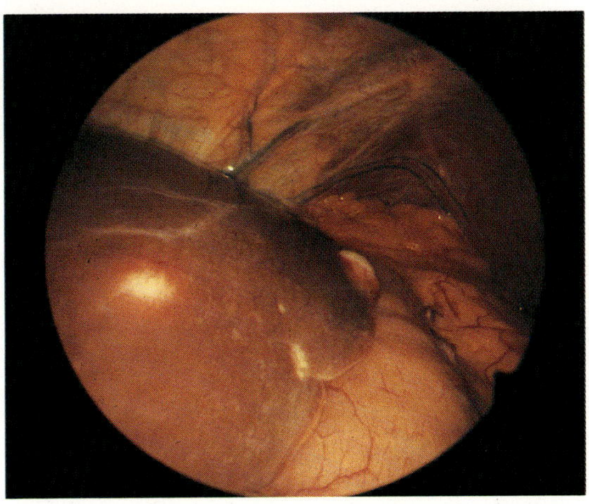

of screening laparoscopy before undertaking hepatic resections for metastatic disease. The sensitivity of available scanning techniques can not pick up these small lesions. The author recommends laparoscopy before angiography because the complication rate with the former is less than with the latter.

Case 4.31

A 64-year-old male 2 years status post-esophagogastrectomy for carcinoma of the stomach presented with weakness. As part of the workup, a CT scan revealed a metastatic lesion in the right lobe of the liver. The rest of the evaulation was normal. Laparoscopic view of the lateral aspect of the right lobe demonstrated an umbilicated metastatic deposit near the dome of the right lobe. There are several 1-mm deposits as well. Also, note diaphragmatic involvement. Dx: Metastatic adenocarcinoma of gastric origin. The umbilicated appearance of metastatic deposits is typical of a gastrointestinal primary. The presence of parietal peritoneal spread was unexpected and probably has prognostic significance. In the author's opinion, oncologists would have a better understanding of the specific stage of disease in many cases if laparoscopy was used more often.

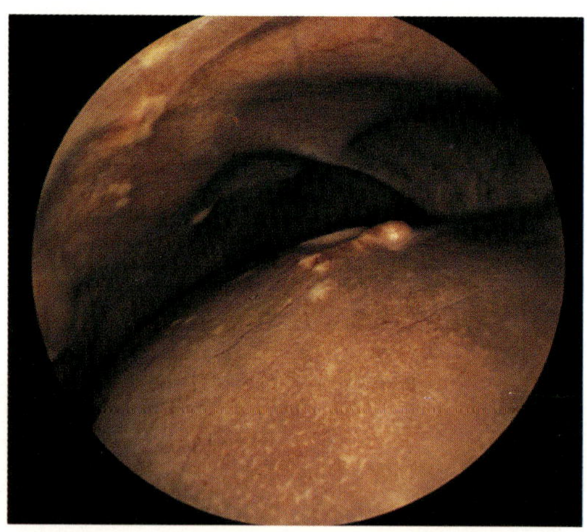

Case 4.32

A 62-year-old female presented with night fevers and anorexia. CT scan revealed mild retroperitoneal lymphadenopathy. There was no peripheral adenopathy, and the bone marrow was nondiagnostic. Percutaneous liver biopsy was also nondiagnostic. Laparoscopic view of the right upper quadrant demonstrated a whitish nodule on the undersurface of the right lobe. The gallbladder is paler than normal and is consistent with chronic cholecystitis. The omentum and small intestine are normal. Dx: Hodgkin's lymphoma. The differential was between Hodgkin's and non-Hodgkin's lymphoma. This 8-mm lesion was not identified on pre-laparoscopy scanning. If a focal nodule were not found, several directed biopsies of the liver would have been taken. If these were negative, open laparotomy would have been performed to obtain a tissue diagnosis. A laparotomy was not necessary in this patient as the liver biopsy was diagnostic.

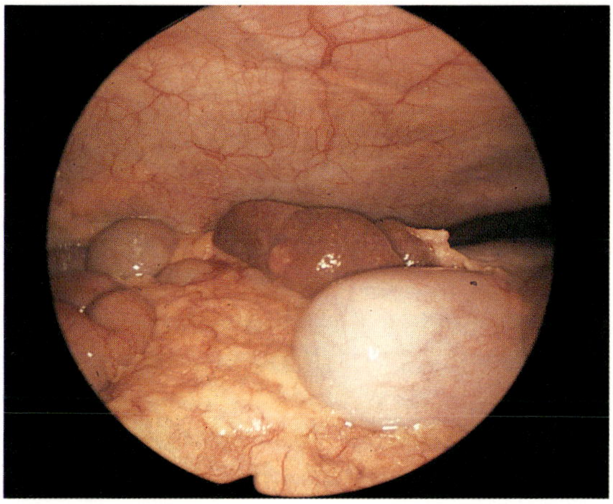

Case 4.33

A 68-year-old female 10 years status post-bilateral mastectomy for carcinoma presented with increasing abdominal girth. A workup revealed a left ovarian mass, ascites, and defects in both lobes of the liver. Laparoscopic view of the lateral segment of the left lobe showed macronodular

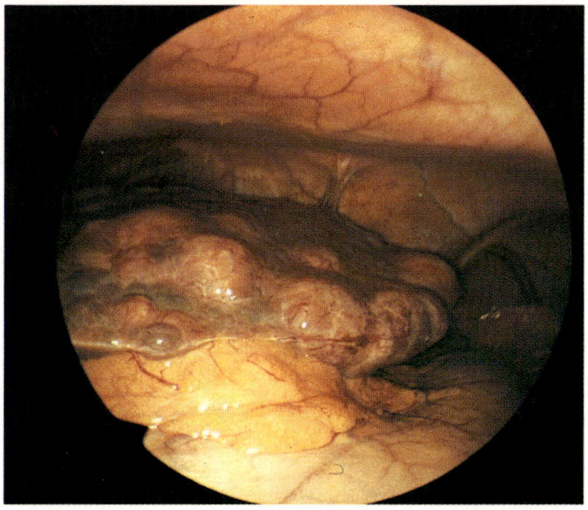

cirrhosis and multiple whitish-red raised metastatic deposits. The diaphragm is in the background. Dx: Metastatic breast carcinoma. Percutaneous blind liver biopsy is contraindicated in the presence of ascites. Laparoscopy is amply suitable in this situation. The original diagnosis of ovarian carcinoma was disproved as a direct result of the laparoscopic findings. Several tissue samples were obtained so that hormonal receptors could be measured.

Case 4.34

A 60-year-old male 1 year status post-right colon resection for carcinoma developed a rising CEA that prompted a CT scan. A defect in the right lobe was seen, and percutaneous blind biopsy was performed that was nondiagnostic. Laparoscopy could not visualize the right lobe because of adhesions. This laparoscopic view of the lateral segment of the left lobe demonstrates a small metastatic deposit next to the falciform ligament. Dx: Metastatic colon carcinoma. This is another clear demonstration of unresectability as determined by laparoscopic findings. This patient already had arteriography in preparation for exploration and resection. This 6-mm lesion could not have been defined by any other modality short of open laparotomy.

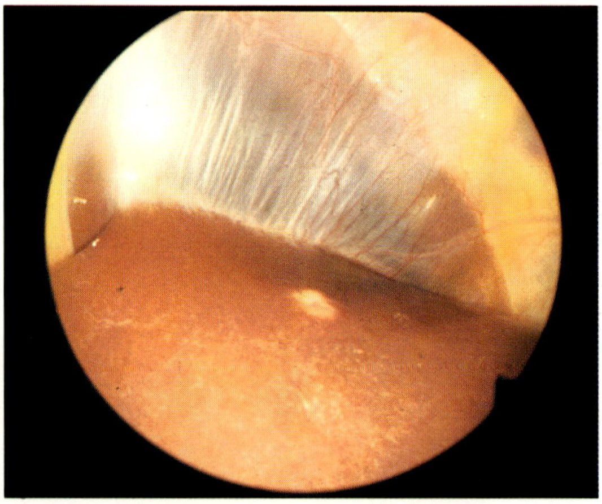

Case 4.35

A 47-year-old male 4 years status post-right thoracotomy and lobectomy for adenocarcinoma presented with increasing abdominal girth. The paracentesis was exudative with negative cytology. CT scan revealed multiple defects in the liver. Laparoscopic view of the right lobe demonstrated a significant amount of metastatic disease not only in the liver but also in the omentum and on the undersurface of the diaphragm. Dx: Adenocarcinoma of lung origin. This patient was thought to have had a curative resection. The presence of ascites precluded a blind percutaneous approach to the liver biopsy. As the histology in the liver was identical to that in the resected lung, no further workup was undertaken. Despite aggressive chemotherapy, he died 2 months after the diagnosis was made.

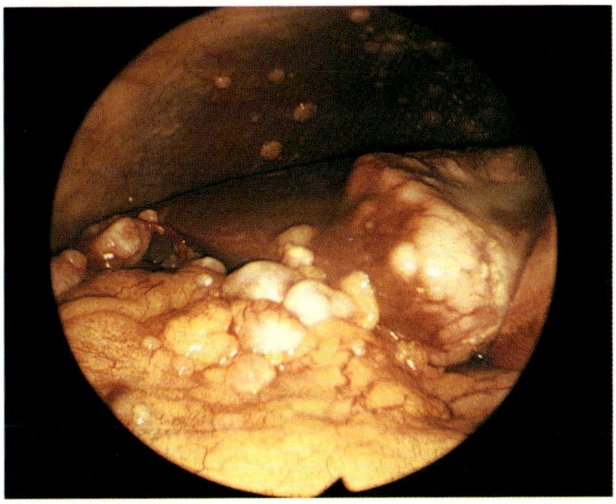

Case 4.36

A 45-year-old female presented with weight loss. The workup included a CT scan that demonstrated a mass in the tail of the pancreas and a defect in the left lobe of the liver. Skinny needle aspiration of the pancreas was nondiagnostic. Laparoscopic view of the lateral segment of the left lobe showed a single, raised metastatic lesion in a slightly prominent

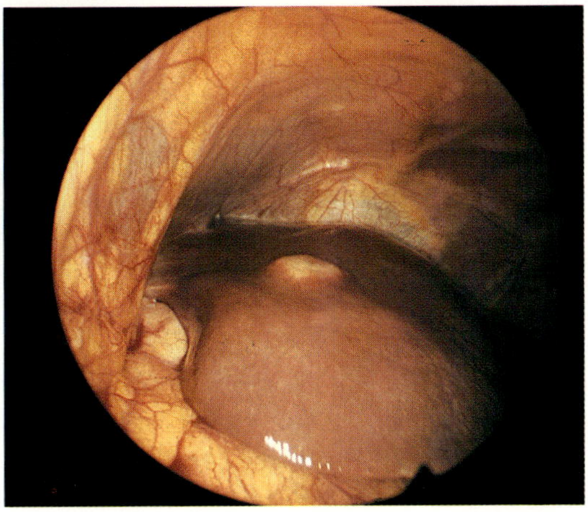

liver segment. The diaphragm is in the *background,* and the falciform ligament is on the *far left.* Dx: Adenocarcinoma consistent with pancreatic origin.

Most gastroenterologists will not perform blind percutaneous liver biopsy of a nonpalpable lesion in the lateral segment of the left lobe, as the segment is usually thin, and the stomach is directly underneath. This is ideal for directed biopsy under visual control with laparoscopy. This patient had a rapidly progressive downhill course. Chemotherapy was offered because of her age but without result.

Case 4.37

A 60-year-old female presented with jaundice and increasing abdominal girth. The workup revealed ascites and multiple defects in both lobes of the liver. Percutaneous blind biopsy was negative, and paracentesis was nondiagnostic as well. Laparoscopic view of the left lobe demonstrated multiple metastatic deposits in a cholestatic liver. The falciform ligament is at the *top,* and the stomach is in the *foreground.* Dx: Undifferentiated carcinoma, primary unknown.

This case is a good demonstration of left lobe pathology causing the lateral segment to be lifted off the stomach. There is always pathology involved when this is seen laparoscopically. In this case, the process is secondary to large metastatic deposits.

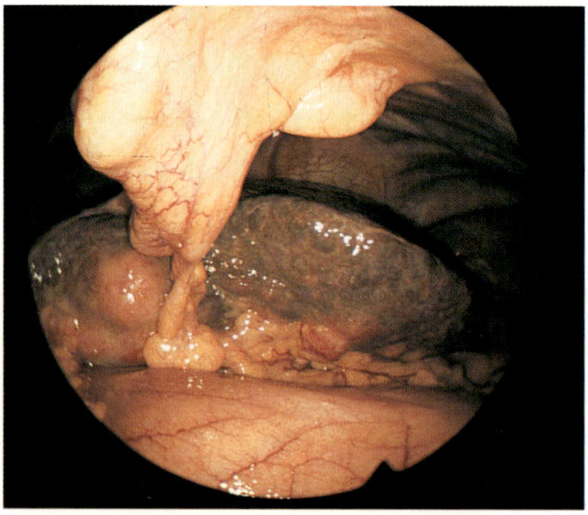

Case 4.38*A–C*

A 68-year-old female presented with weight loss. The workup was negative, except for the CT scan, which revealed multiple filling defects in both lobes of the liver (Fig. 4.38**A**). Percutaneous blind liver biopsy was

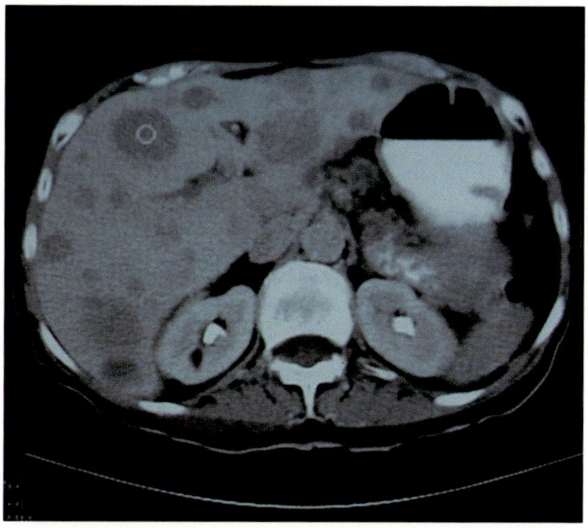

A

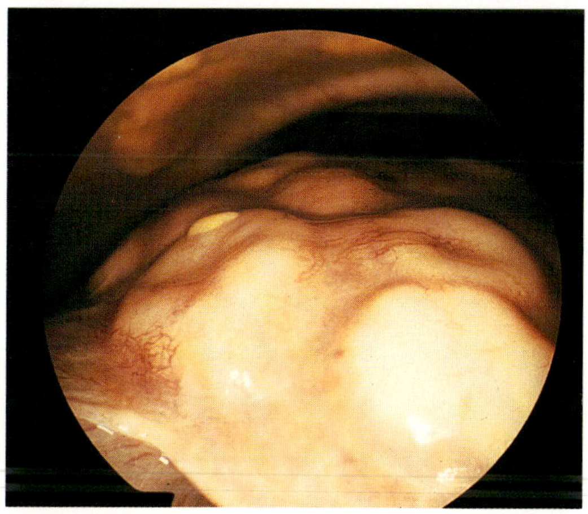

B

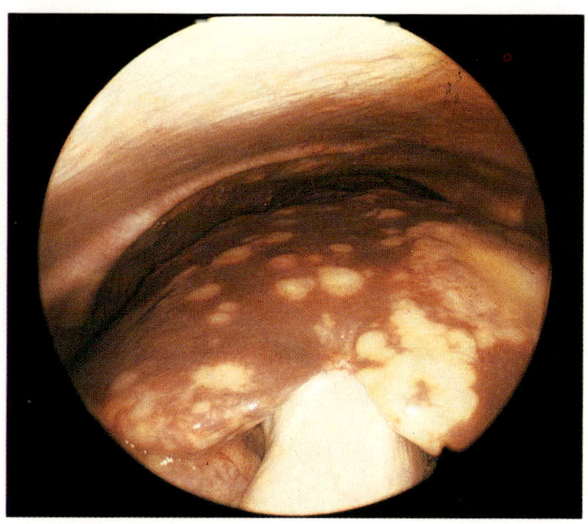

C

negative. A repeat percutaneous biopsy was also negative. Laparoscopic view of the right lobe revealed multiple metastatic deposits as shown in this closeup view (Fig. 4.38**B**). Neovascularization is evident. Dx: Adenocarcinoma primary unknown.

The author is always amazed when blind percutaneous biopsy is negative in cases in which there is so much disease present. Figure 6.38**C** is a different patient with metastatic pancreatic carcinoma in whom percutaneous biopsy was tried first and failed. In patients who have this much disease, percutaneous biopsy is a reasonable choice, as the incidence of a false-negative result will be low, but not as low as a directed biopsy via laparoscopy.

Case 4.39

A 78-year-old female 2 years status post-excisional surgery for ovarian carcinoma presented with jaundice. A sonogram showed markedly dilated intrahepatic ducts with multiple areas consistent with metastatic disease. CT scan was equivocal regarding metastatic disease. There was no ascitic fluid present. Laparoscopic view of a markedly cholestatic liver with multiple areas of metastatic disease is shown. The round ligament separating the medial segment from the lateral segment of the left lobe is clearly seen. Dx: Metastatic ovarian carcinoma with psammoma bodies.

It is distinctly unusual for ovarian carcinoma to be metastatic to the liver without peritoneal spread and ascites. There is nothing diagnostic in terms of the appearance of the ovarian carcinoma in the liver, which is why biopsy is mandatory for any lesion in which a definitive diagnosis is necessary.

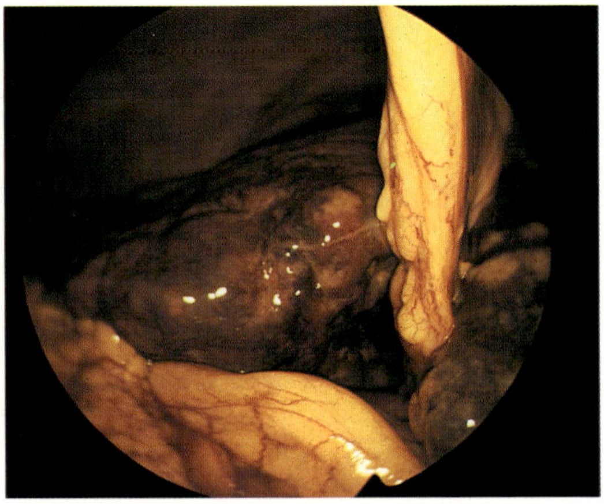

Case 4.40

A 60-year-old female presented with right upper quadrant discomfort and a palpable mass. A sonogram demonstrated a thickened gallbladder, gallstones, and several masses in the right lobe near the gallbladder. Laparoscopic view of the gallbladder and medial segment of the left lobe is shown. There is a whitish plaque present at the dome of the gallbladder that could only be seen after the omental adhesion was lifted off by the second puncture probe. There are several metastatic lesions in the medial segment. The first portion of the duodenum is visible in the *foreground.* Dx: Carcinoma of the gallbladder. The gallbladder is easily seen with laparoscopy, and carcinomatous change can be detected if the visceral peritoneal surface of the gallbladder is involved. If a biopsy of the gallbladder wall is taken, the author has found the lancet-shaped biopsy forceps to be very useful in obtaining tangential biopsies.

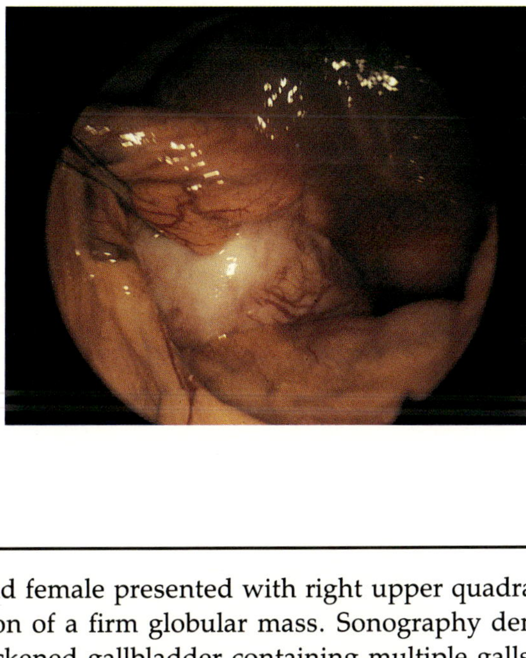

Case 4.41

An 82-year-old female presented with right upper quadrant discomfort and suggestion of a firm globular mass. Sonography demonstrated an enlarged, thickened gallbladder containing multiple gallstones suggestive of carcinoma. Laparoscopic view of the gallbladder demonstrated two small nodules at the dome near the end of the palpating probe. Although it can not be appreciated in this figure, the gallbladder wall was very firm to probe palpation. The hepatic flexure is in the background. Dx: Carcinoma of the gallbladder. The nodules yielded the positive biopsy, but the clinical appearance was one of total involvement. Considering the patient's advanced age and other medical problems, surgery was not recommended.

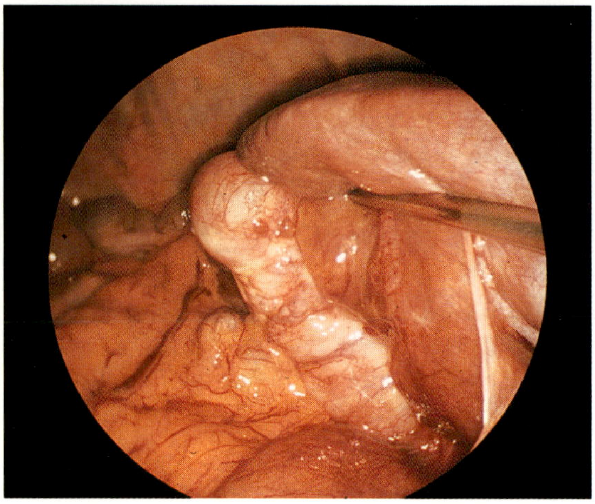

Case 4.42

A 56-year-old male presented with an asymptomatic mass in the right upper quadrant. The workup was negative, except for a CT scan that showed a defect in the medial segment of the left lobe. Incidental gallstones were noted. Laparoscopic view of the gallbladder demonstrated subperitoneal involvement by carcinoma on the medial side of the gallbladder. The marked prominence of the medial segment of the left lobe is secondary to a subcapsular metastatic deposit. Dx: Adenocarcinoma of the gallbladder with metastatic liver disease. A tangential biopsy of the firm and whitish area of the medial aspect of the gallbladder was positive for adenocarcinoma of biliary tract origin. The author was surprised to see such a large metastatic deposit when not all of the gallbladder was as yet involved with carcinoma. One can still see a "robin's egg blue" color to the dome of the gallbladder.

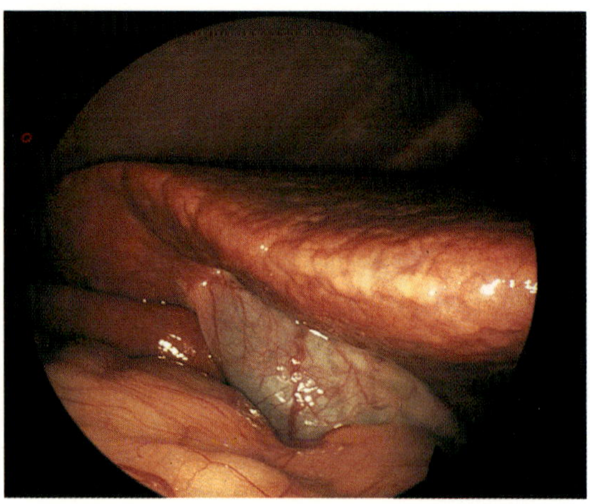

Case 4.43

A 54-year-old male with a known history of hepatitis B presented with worsening of his liver function tests. CT scan was included as part of his workup, which demonstrated several defects in both lobes that were similar to those from a previous scan performed 3 years before. The alpha-fetoprotein was slightly elevated. Laparoscopic view of the left lobe showed multiple tumor masses in a cirrhotic liver. The liver is lifted off the stomach by the infiltrative process in the liver. The lesser omentum is clearly seen between the liver and the stomach. The diaphragm is in the *background.* Dx: Hepatoma. Laparoscopy demonstrated a much more extensive process than the CT scan seemed to show. Clearly, this patient was not a candidate for any resectional therapy. Directed biopsy was straightforward. This patient had a rapidly progressive downhill course.

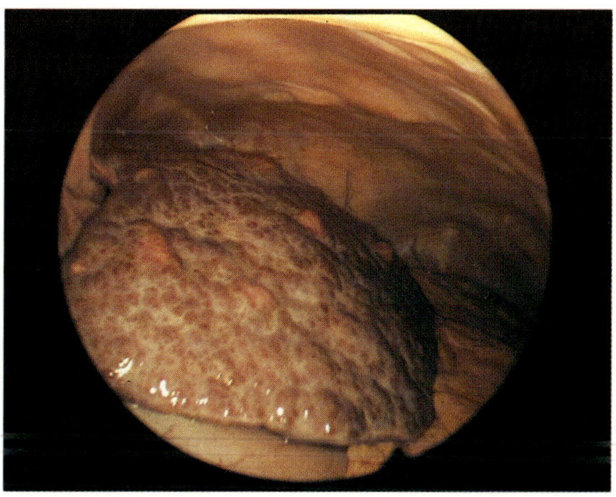

Case 4.44

A 57-year-old male with a 15-year history of biopsy-proven eosinophilic gastritis presented with weight loss, upper GI bleeding, and abnormal liver function tests (LFT). CT scan demonstrated multiple defects in the liver and a moderate amount of ascites. Laparoscopic view of the left lobe showed several metastatic deposits in the lateral segment of the left lobe near the falciform ligament. There is a modest amount of congestion in the liver as manifested by the rounded liver edge and by the purplish color of the "normal" liver. The stomach is visible in the *foreground.* Dx: Undifferentiated tumor with histiocytic features. This patient's symptoms were underestimated because of the underlying eosinophilic gastritis. As a result, an advanced disease state was found at the time of laparoscopy. The directed biposy was straightforward.

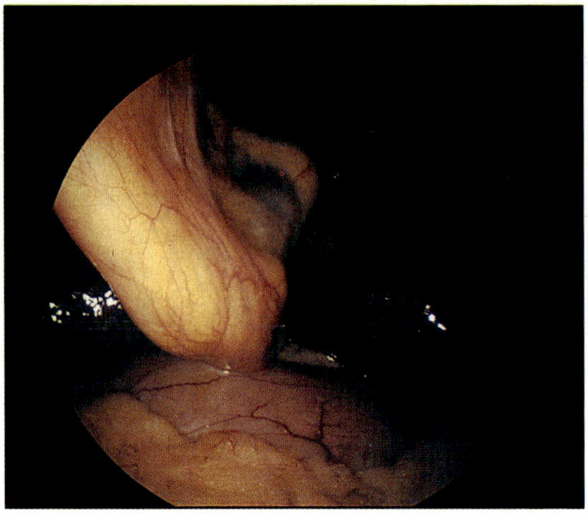

Case 4.45

A 68-year-old female presented with weight loss and the recent onset of diabetes. A workup showed abnormal LFTs, which prompted a CT scan. Several defects were noted in the right lobe of the liver, and a thickened pancreatic body was identified. Laparoscopic view of the right lobe of the liver demonstrated a large metastatic deposit just superior to the gallbladder. A smaller lesion is faintly visible in the background. Dx: Adenocarcinoma consistent with pancreatic primary. Carcinoma of the body of the pancreas usually presents late in its clinical course. The gallbladder is not distended. There was some consideration given to a gallbladder primary based on the CT scan. It is understandable as one sees the close relationship of the gallbladder to the metastatic deposit.

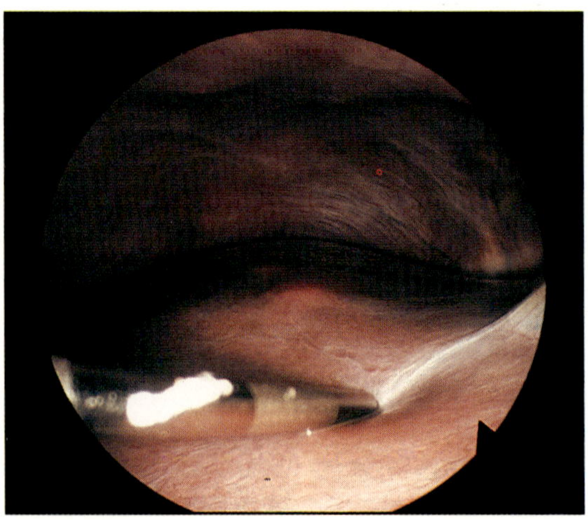

Case 4.46

A 71-year-old male presented with anorexia and weight loss. During the workup a CT scan revealed a defect in the right lobe of the liver. An evaluation of the gastrointestinal tract was unrewarding. Laparoscopic view of the left lobe demonstrated a significant metastatic deposit on the anterior aspect of the lateral segment with a smaller satellite lesion to its left. There is a wedge-shaped defect in the center of the lesion with a blood clot present. This is the biopsy site. Dx: Adenocarcinoma primary unknown. When there is a superficial deposit without a deeper component, CT may not visualize it, as in this patient. Notice the normal juxtaposition of the lateral segment of the liver and the stomach wall. After every liver biopsy, a good blood clot should be seen laparoscopically, such as is seen in this case. The primary was never identified.

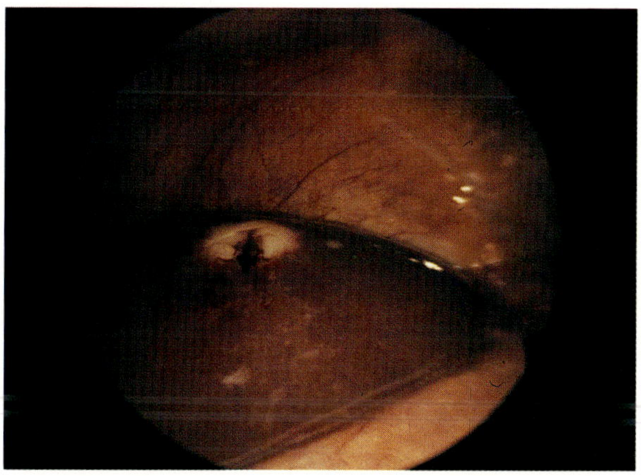

Case 4.47

A 47-year-old female presented with weight loss, left upper abdominal pain, and an enlarging abdomen. Physical examination revealed a mass in the left upper quadrant of the abdomen. CT scan demonstrated a large retroperitoneal mass and several defects in both lobes of the liver. Laparoscopic view of the right upper quadrant showed a yellowish, metastatic lesion on the edge of the medial segment of the left lobe of the liver. The palpating probe is elevating the liver. The gallbladder, hepatic flexure of the colon, and first portion of the duodenum are visualized and are normal. Dx: Adenocarcinoma of adrenal cortex origin. In this patient, laparoscopy not only made the diagnosis but also proved non-resectability as well. In the author's experience, this double benefit is not uncommon when dealing with metastatic liver disease. In many cases, other invasive tests, such as angiograms, frequently are not needed. This patient failed to respond to aggressive chemotherapy.

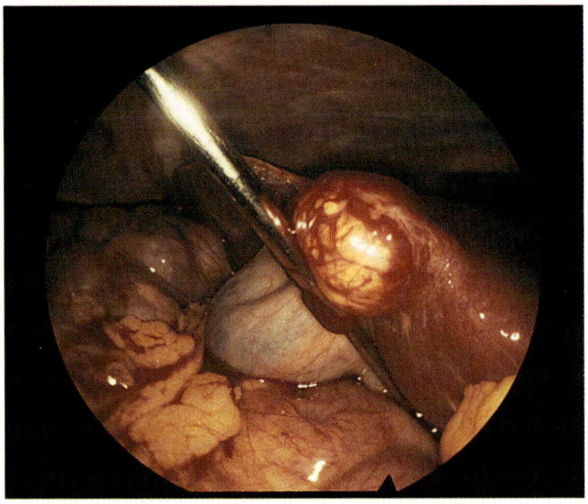

5

ASCITES

Ascites of unknown etiology is a relatively common indication for laparoscopy. Surgeons are frequently called on to perform paracentesis for both diagnostic and therapeutic reasons. A natural extension is laparoscopy. Laparoscopy is indicated for exudative ascites usually, as transudative ascites is almost always on the basis of a "medical" disease that is often diagnosed without invasive measures. Not infrequently, a definitive diagnosis is not possible on examination of the paracentesis fluid. Cytological examination, when positive, usually precludes the need for further diagnostic steps, but if negative, does not rule in or out malignant disease. It is in just this setting that laparoscopy has great value.

Laparoscopy can not be performed with tense ascites. Significant reduction of the ascitic fluid is necessary before attempting the procedure. This is accomplished by placing a 5F multiholed polyethylene indwelling peritoneal catheter for 24 to 48 hr beforehand. With exudative ascites, rapid decompression may proceed without fear of renal complications. This is not the case with transudative ascites, and extreme care must be taken. The laparoscopic puncture must be placed significantly higher on the abdominal wall, as the abdomen is ptotic, and visualization of the liver may be difficult if a standard or lower incision is made. Both benign and, more frequently, malignant causes are found laparoscopically. The fact that most cases will not be amenable to surgical therapy should not detract from the diagnostic accuracy that in the author's experience approaches 95%.

BENIGN

Case 5.1

A 65-year-old male with recent onset of exudative ascites. The past history was noncontributory, and all blood tests, including liver function tests, were normal. CT scan showed no abnormality except ascites. Laparoscopic view of macronodular cirrhosis is shown. Ascitic fluid level is visible in the *background*. Note the prominent quadrate lobe and the pale gallbladder typical of cirrhosis. The colon to the *left* and the stomach to the *right* show no obvious signs of portal hypertension. Directed liver biopsy: Cirrhosis.

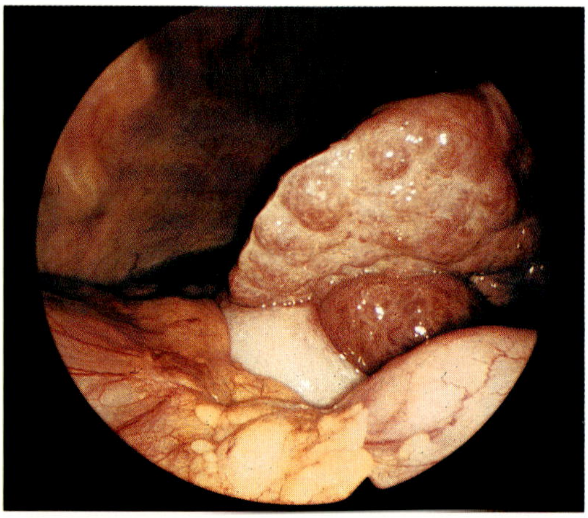

Case 5.2

A 37-year-old male without history of alcohol abuse presented with recent onset of tense ascites. The patient had exposure to industrial chemicals. All other workup was nonrevealing, with the exception of exudative ascites. Laparoscopic view of the right lobe of the liver is shown. Ascitic fluid level is visible in the *background*. Pale gallbladder is visible in the *foreground*. Liver capsule is somewhat fibrotic. Very early regeneration of the liver is evident by its "bumpy" appearance. Directed liver biopsy: Cirrhosis. Cases 5.1 and 5.2 demonstrate the uncommon need of laparoscopy for benign liver disease. Although cirrhosis was unexpected from the preoperative evaluation, it is the most common cause of nonmalignant ascites. Massive ascites is a contraindication to blind percutaneous biopsy, because of fear of dislodging the clot at the biopsy site. Laparoscopy is the safest and most accurate way to obtain tissue for histological diagnosis in this setting. The ease with which biopsy can be obtained is evident from the laparoscopic photographs.

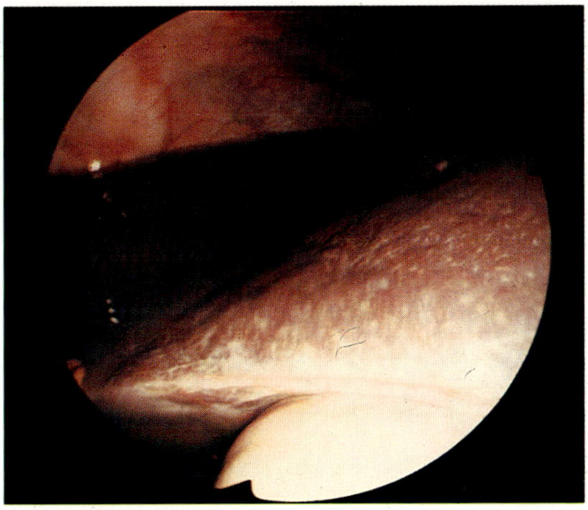

Case 5.3

A 40-year-old female 2 years status post-kidney transplant for end-stage renal disease secondary to diabetes mellitus. The patient developed recent tense ascites that contained a high lymphocyte count. The kidney function was excellent. A mild elevation of the alkaline phosphatase was present. Rest of the workup was unrewarding. Laparoscopic view of an

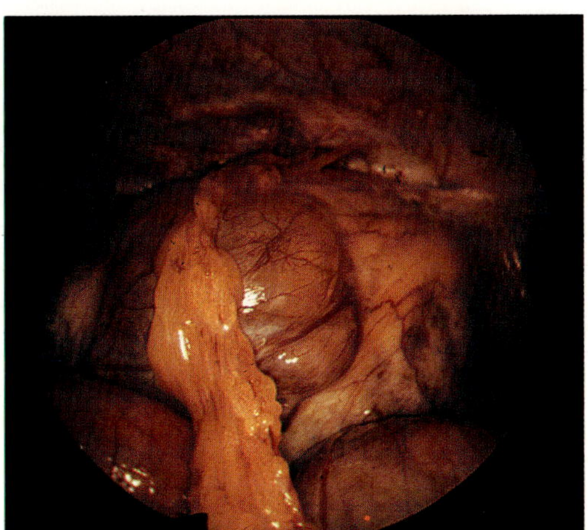

unexpected leaking lymphocele around the transplant in the right iliac fossa. Omental adhesions on the right lateral abdominal wall were an incidental finding. The small intestine is in the *foreground,* and it is normal. The preoperative diagnosis in case 5-3 was thought most likely to be tuberculous peritonitis, as the patient was on steroids and the lymphocyte count of the exudative ascitic fluid was elevated. The finding of a leaking lymphocele surrounding the transplant is unusual. The transplant was eventually removed. The patient received another donor kidney, but postoperative sepsis resulted in mortality. Nevertheless, laparoscopy was instrumental in making the diagnosis.

Case 5.4

A 66-year-old male with recent onset of ascites and weight loss. The patient had chronic renal failure based on hypertensive nephropathy and severe gouty tophus arthritis. Peritoneal tap revealed abundant mesothelial cells and lymphocytes. Laparoscopic view of exudate in the left upper quadrant with multiple soft, whitish nodules present on the small bowel loop in the *foreground* and on the parietal peritoneum on the *right.* Ascitic fluid is seen over the small bowel loop. Directed biopsy revealed caseating granulomata. Diagnosis: Tuberculous peritonitis.

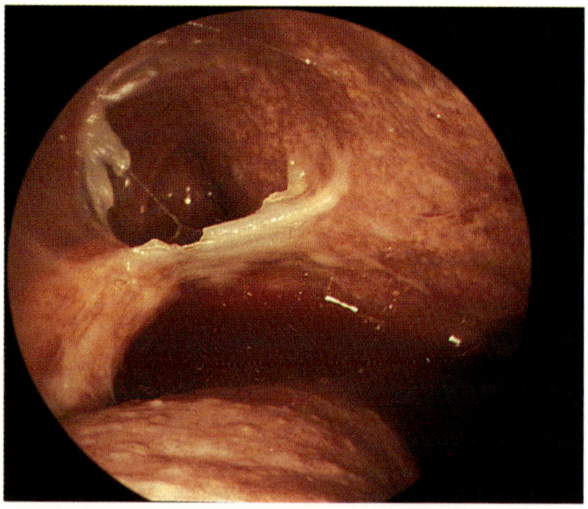

Case 5.5

A 38-year-old Filipino male with recent ascites, weight loss, and low grade fevers. The workup was negative, except for atypical lymphocytes on the peritoneal tap. Laparoscopy revealed multiple fine, whitish nodules on the parietal peritoneum *(background)* and on the small intestine *(foreground)*. Directed biopsy: Tuberculous peritonitis. Cases 5.4 and 5.5 demonstrate the typical findings of peritoneal tuberculosis. It is impossible to establish the difference between malignant disease and tuberculous disease based on the macroscopic appearance alone. Biopsy is mandatory. The presence of granulomata or the actual bacillus confirms the diagnosis. Treatment should be initiated before culture confirmation occurs. The author recommends the use of a narrow laparoscope (3 or 5 mm in diameter) when tuberculous peritonitis is suspected to decrease the risk of bowel perforation. The lancet-shaped biopsy forceps is an ideal instrument for taking tangential biopsies from the bowel wall itself. Laparoscopy is the procedure of choice when tuberculous peritonitis is suspected.

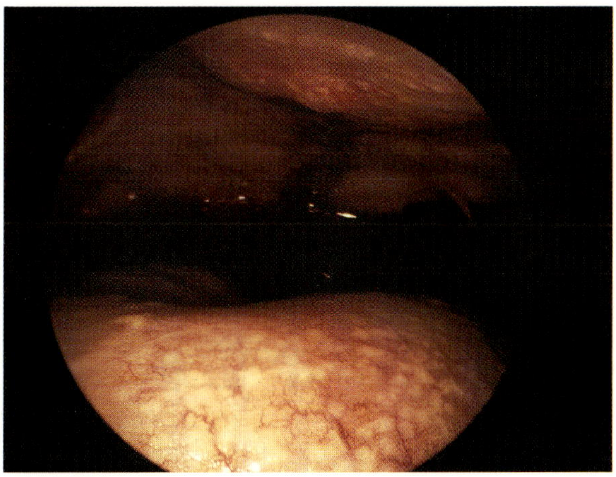

MALIGNANT

Case 5.6

A 65-year-old female with known pseudomyxomatous ovarian carcinoma developed tense ascites with multiple encapsulated pseudomyxomatous deposits. Laparoscopic view inside a large encysted metastatic deposit is shown. The gelatinous nature of the ascites is readily apparent. Case 5.6 illustrates an unusual and difficult case for laparoscopy. Multiple attempts at percutaneous paracentesis failed in decompression of the encysted deposits. The laparoscope was used as a therapeutic modality here. A second puncture trocar (5-mm) was placed into the "cyst," and active suction was required to remove the tenacious material. The rather dramatic relief of the obstructive component was rapid. This patient required multiple aspirations over a period of 3 years before her death.

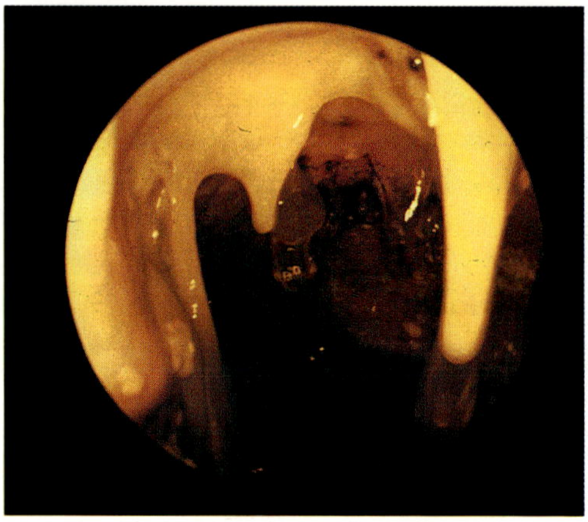

Case 5.7

A 67-year-old female with rapidly accumulating ascites. Paracentesis revealed an exudative ascites with atypical cells. An extensive evaluation was nondiagnostic. Laparoscopy showed multiple whitish plaque-like deposits on the parietal peritoneal surface. The round ligament in this picture was typical of the rest of the abdominal peritoneal cavity. Biopsy: Signet-ring carcinoma. After this surprise finding at laparoscopy, the patient underwent upper gastrointestinal endoscopy. A small primary was identified in the cardia of the stomach. The previous UGI series was reviewed and still found to be negative. In the author's experience, it is rare not to obtain histological proof of the diagnosis in malignant ascites.

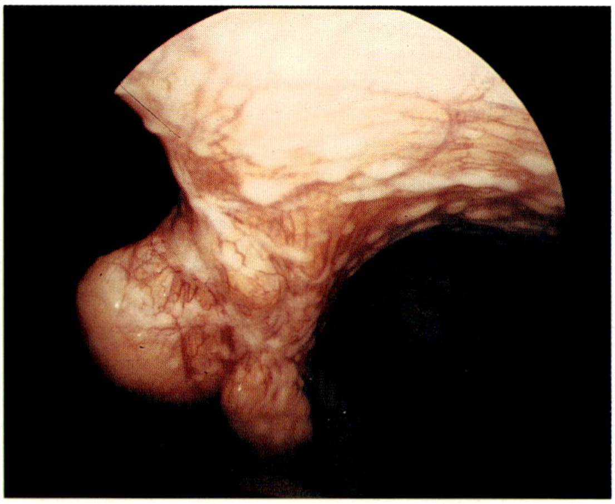

Case 5.8

A 65-year-old male with known asbestos exposure presented with increasing abdominal girth. Chest radiographs were unremarkable. Paracentesis revealed mesothelial cells. Laparoscopic view of the anterior parietal peritoneal surface just below the umbilicus. The parietal peritoneum is replaced by an infiltrating tumor. Biopsy: Primary peritoneal mesothelioma.

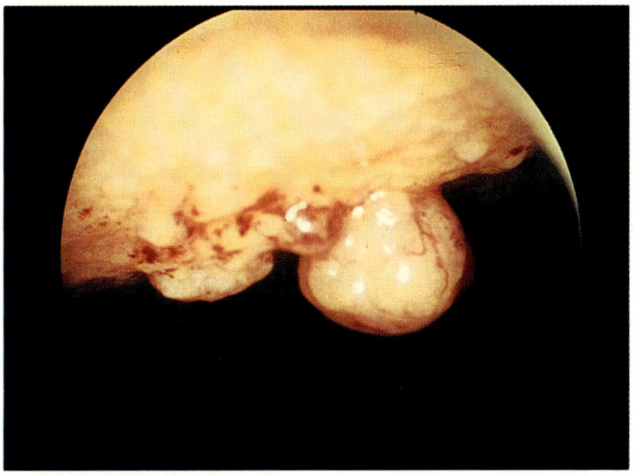

Case 5.9

A 25-year-old male jewelry worker went for routine inguinal hernia repair. The pathology report of the hernia sac was consistent with mesothelioma. This patient was asymptomatic. Laparoscopy was per-

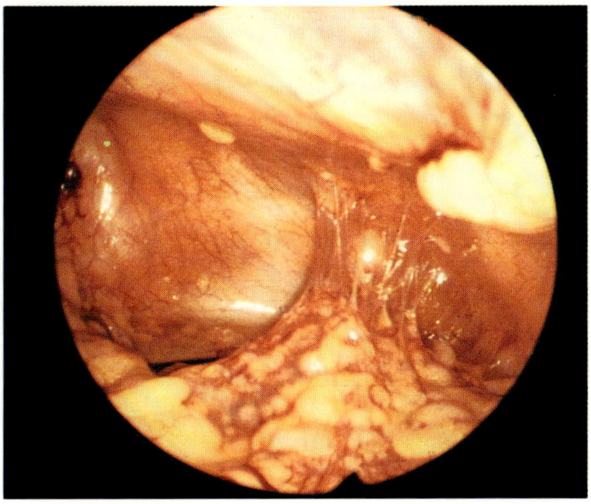

formed for confirmation. Laparoscopic view showing the omentum and lower pelvic parietal peritoneum infiltrated by a friable, fleshy tumor. Note that the omentum adhered to the internal inguinal ring closure site. A small amount of ascitic fluid is present in the lower left corner of the picture. Biopsy: Mesothelioma. Cases 5.8 and 5.9 demonstrate why laparoscopy is the procedure of choice for primary peritoneal diseases. Direct inspection of almost all of the parietal surface is accomplished by laparoscopy. Directed biopsy is easily performed. It is usually not necessary to inject local anesthesia directly into the biopsy site if tumor is present. However, if relatively normal parietal peritoneum is in the jaws of the biopsy forceps, application of local anesthesia before biopsy occurs is appropriate. In the case of mesothelioma, cytological examination of the ascitic fluid is frequently nondiagnostic.

Case 5.10

A 56-year-old male oriental with rapidly increasing abdominal distention. The patient had a known history of alcohol abuse with worsening of liver function. Paracentesis revealed bloody ascites. Urgent laparoscopy showed diffuse hepatocellular carcinoma involving both lobes of the liver. The left lobe is seen with obvious infiltration. Bloody ascites is present. Directed biopsy: Hepatocellular carcinoma. Bloody ascites is usually indicative of malignant disease in the absence of trauma. Although the diagnosis of hepatocellular carcinoma was expected preoperatively, urgent laparoscopy was performed to determine whether a remedial situation existed and to obtain a tissue diagnosis.

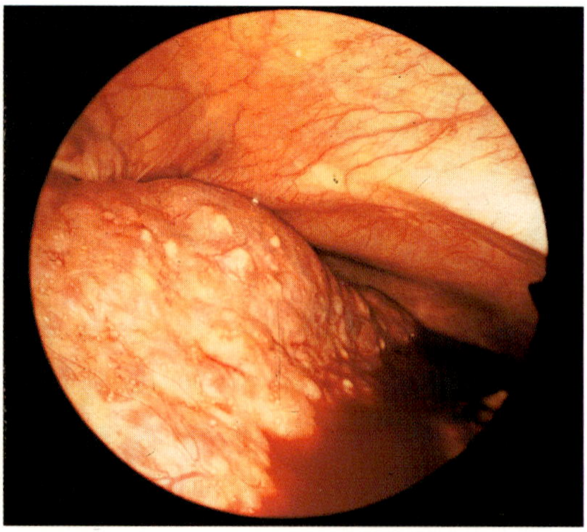

Case 5.11

A 40-year-old female presented with new onset ascites. Workup, including pelvic exam and CT scan, was negative for primary disease. Laparoscopic view of the right hemidiaphragm and the right lobe of the liver with multiple whitish plaques on the parietal peritoneum and right hemidiaphragm is shown *(background)*. Ascites is present over the right lobe. Biopsy: Adenocarcinoma with psammoma bodies.

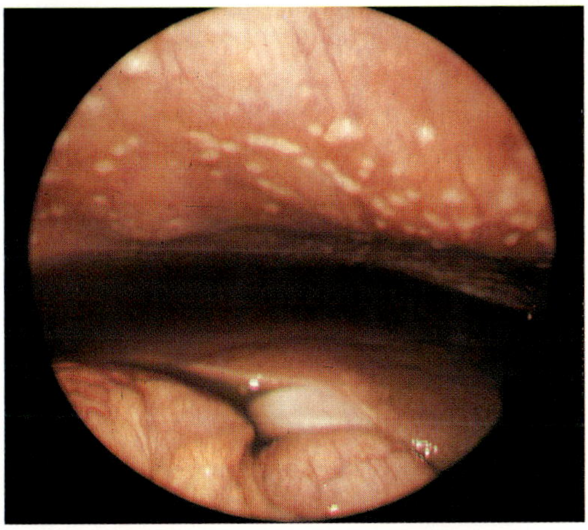

Case 5.12

A 69-year-old female presented with recent ascites. Workup was negative. Laparoscopy showed an omental cake. Blood is noted at the biopsy site. Biopsy: Adenocarcinoma with psammoma bodies.

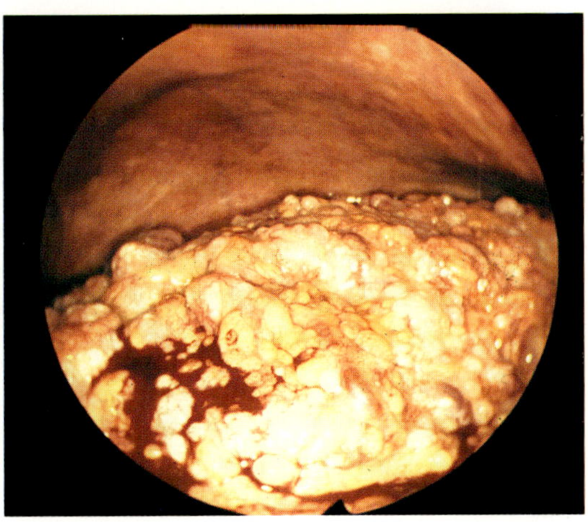

Case 5.13

A 50-year-old female presented with recent onset of ascites. Laparoscopic view of a contracted omentum infiltrating the abdominal wall is shown. Several smaller metastatic deposits are visible on the anterior parietal peritoneum. Biopsy: Adenocarcinoma consistent with gynecological primary. Cases 5.11, 5.12, and 5.13 illustrate unsuspected ovarian carcinoma. All of these patients were thoroughly evaluated before laparoscopy by means of pelvic exam and either CT scan or sonography. Each patient had paracentesis that showed exudative ascites. The point must be made that if ovarian carcinoma is suspected preoperatively, laparoscopy is not indicated. There have been case reports of implantation of carcinoma at the laparoscopic insertion site after surgical debulking and cure by chemotherapy. However, in the face of no objective evidence of pelvic disease, laparoscopy should be performed. Two of these patients required extended paracentesis to adequately decompress the ascitic fluid in order to allow visualization with the laparoscope.

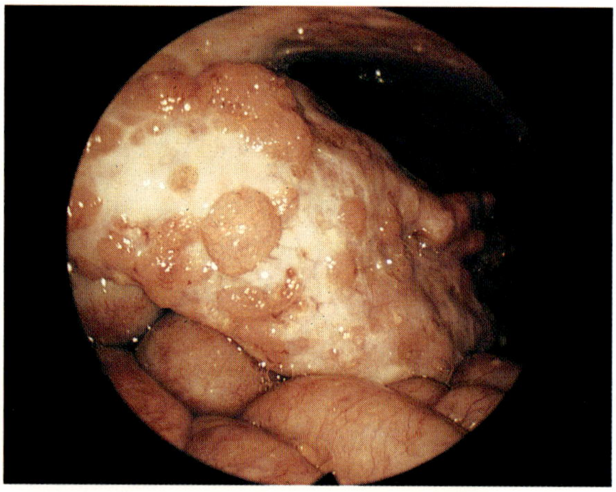

Case 5.14

A 55-year-old female 15 years status post-mastectomy for carcinoma presented with recent ascites. Abdominal CT scan was negative with the exception of ascites. Laparoscopy demonstrated multiple soft, whitish deposits on multiple loops of small intestine. Biopsy: Metastatic breast carcinoma.

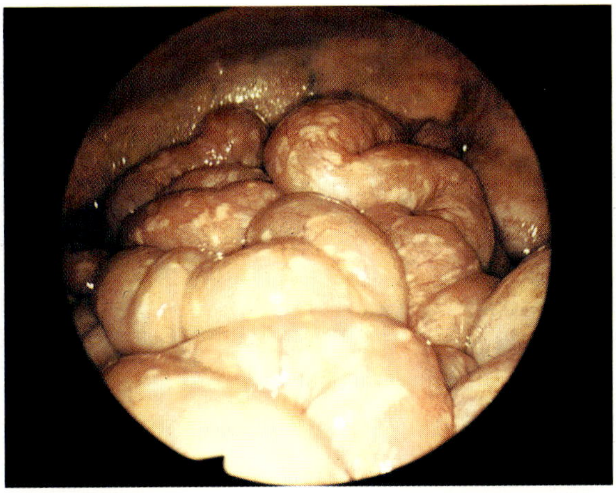

Case 5.15

A 65-year-old female 10 years status post-mastectomy with recent onset of ascites. Laparoscopic view of omentum infiltrated by tumor. The liver was clear. Several loops of small intestine are visible in the background. Biopsy: Omentum infiltrated by metastatic breast carcinoma. Surgeons are familiar with the occasional long delay in the presentation of metastatic breast disease. Cases 5.14 and 5.15 demonstrate this clearly. Extreme care must be taken in obtaining serosal biopsies of intestinal viscera, as in case 5.14. The author has found the lancet-shaped biopsy forceps to be ideal for this type of biopsy. Proper staging of breast carcinoma is mandatory for the appropriate chemotherapeutic management. Cytology on these patients was nondiagnostic. Histological proof of the primary was ascertained by the directed biospy.

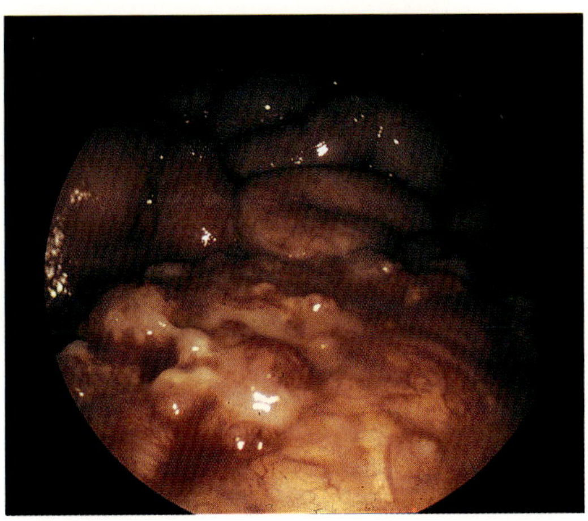

Case 5.16

A 65-year-old female 25 years status post-abdominoperineal resection for adenocarcinoma of the rectum presented with recent onset of ascites. The noninvasive workup was negative. Laparoscopic view of the left upper quadrant reveals several small whitish metastatic lesions on the surface of the left hemidiaphragm. There is a moderate amount of ascitic fluid visible in the *background* with omentum floating in the fluid. The left lobe of the liver, stomach, and transverse colon are visible in the *foreground,* and they are normal. Directed lancet-shaped biopsy of the lesions revealed adenocarcinoma consistent with an ovarian primary. The pelvis could not be visualized because of extensive adhesion formation from the previous abdominoperineal resection. Even though the preoperative sonogram and CT scan did not reveal the ovarian primary, surgical exploration demonstrated a primary in the left ovary. Appropriate gynecological surgery was undertaken as a direct consequence of the laparoscopic findings. This case further strengthens the concept that laparoscopy is a highly accurate diagnostic modality in exudative ascites.

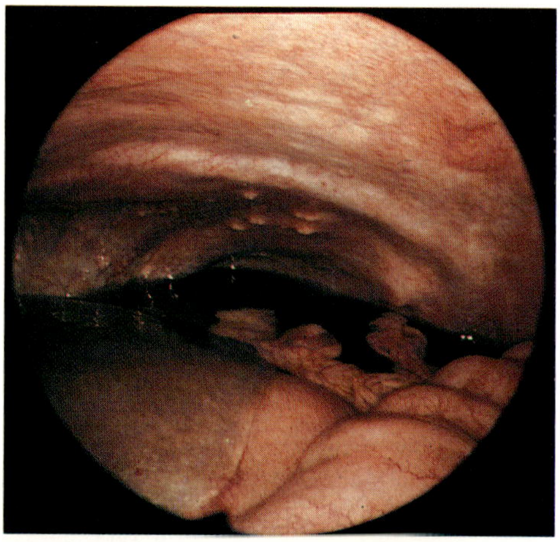

Case 5.17

A 68-year-old male presented with recent onset of an increased abdominal girth. Sonogram and CT scan demonstrated ascites. Multiple attempts at paracentesis were unsuccessful in obtaining fluid for evaluation. Sonographic aspiration yielded turbid exudative fluid with negative cytology. Laparoscopic view of the right lower quadrant showed the parietal peritoneum to be finely granular, suggestive of infiltration. Multiple loops of small bowel are fixed to each other clearly visible in the foreground. Directed biopsy revealed undifferentiated carcinoma. The gross picture was compatible with either infiltration or inflammation. The necessity for histological proof is mandatory, and biopsy should always be obtained. The lancet-shaped biopsy forceps should be utilized in this type of biopsy.

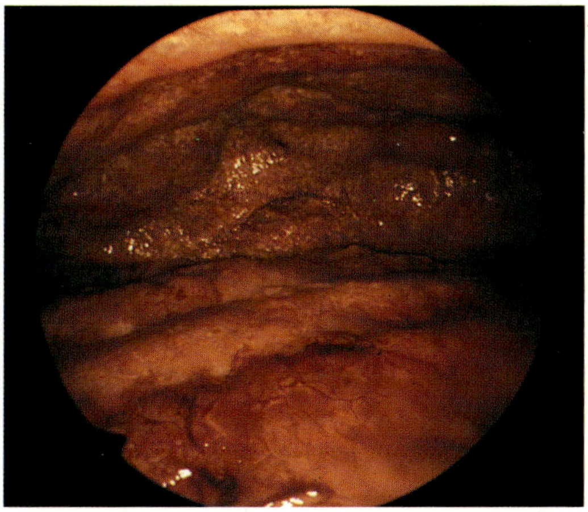

Case 5.18

A 66-year-old female presented with the recent onset of ascites. Upper GI and small bowel series was consistent with either ileitis or tumor infiltration of the small bowel. Paracentesis revealed an exudate with negative cytology. Laparoscopic view of the right lower quadrant shows the omentum to be infiltrated with tumor. The tip of the palpating probe is pointing to a loop of small bowel that is congested secondary to tumor infiltration of the mesentery. There is also metastatic parietal peritoneal disease as well. Omental biopsy showed signet-ring adenocarcinoma. The approach to this patient was dramatically altered by the results of laparoscopy. While the actual diagnosis was proved by the procedure, much more information was gained about the extent of disease. In the author's experience, this is an unusual indication for laparoscopy, as the differential between inflammation and tumor infiltration can almost always be ascertained by relatively noninvasive procedures

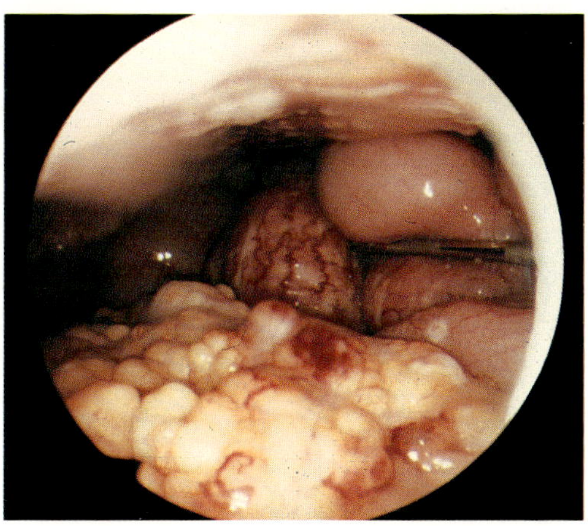

6

THERAPEUTIC LAPAROSCOPY

As most of the gastrointestinal laparoscopies in the United States are performed by gastroenterologists, surgical therapeutic maneuvers via the laparoscope have not progressed as rapidly as diagnostic procedures. This is certainly not the case with the specialty of gynecology, in which laparoscopy plays a prominent role. Also, in many European centers, therapeutic laparoscopic manipulations have become commonplace. As the author gained experience with the many advantages of laparoscopy and as the invasive radiologists began to report therapeutic procedures performed under indirect x-ray control, it became obvious that several surgical problems could be safely dealt with by laparoscopy under direct visualization. Some procedures that the author would have ordinarily performed by laparotomy are now undertaken by laparoscopic surgery. The advantages to the patient are less pain postoperatively, less postoperative ileus, and less time spent on inpatient hospital stays. In the specific cases of chronic abdominal pain secondary to adhesions, the laparoscopic lysis is performed under local anesthesia, which obviates the general anesthetic risk completely. In the more complicated procedures general anesthesia is required. The author hopes that the following pictorial presentations will open the door for more use of the laparoscope for definitive therapy, and that perhaps it will stimulate other newer uses of this exciting technique.

Case 6.1*A–I*

A 22-year-old male with a known amebic abscess in the right lobe of the liver was referred for surgical drainage after failing to resolve with medical therapy. CT scan (Fig. 6.1**A–C**) of the upper abdomen demonstrates an abscess high in the right lobe surrounded by lung. The invasive radiologists were consulted, but they felt that percutaneous drainage would be impossible without penetrating the chest cavity. Laparoscopic drainage was performed under general anesthesia. Figure 6.1**D** shows the in situ appearance of the abscess adherent to the right hemidiaphragm by adhesions. The liver is otherwise normal in appearance. Figure 6.1**E** demonstrates the laparoscopic scissors properly positioned to begin lysis of the adhesions. The adhesions have been lysed with little bleeding (Fig. 6.1**F**). Figure 6.1**G** shows the 18-gauge aspirating needle inserted into the abscess with complete collapse of the abscess cavity. The size of the abscess can be appreciated by the now-visible diaphragm behind the liver. Sixty cubic centimeters of an anchovy paste-like material typical of an amebic abscess were aspirated. The scissors was connected to an electrocautery unit, and the abscess wall was unroofed with minimal bleeding. Figure 6.1**H** reveals the cut surface of the liver parenchyma, and a sterile 10 Fr nasogastric tube, which was inserted into the abscess cavity under direct vision via the original second puncture sleeve, exiting from the liver. The total operative time was 1 hr. Figure 6.1**I** is a sinogram taken on the third post laparoscopic day, demonstrating the size of the abscess cavity and its location near the right hemidiaphragm. This case was attempted laparoscopically with the full understanding that if it could not be performed properly, a laparotomy would be undertaken. All the laparoscopic manipulations were in essence the same as would be performed through a laparotomy incision. There was no compromise in the exposure as can be appreciated by the pictures. The ease of the incision and drainage of the abscess by the laparoscopic approach allowed a surprisingly smooth postoperative course, in that only small amounts of oral pain medications were needed after the first day. The patient was discharged on the 5th day. The abscess resolved completely by the 4th week after drainage, as documented by outpatient sinography, and the drain was removed.

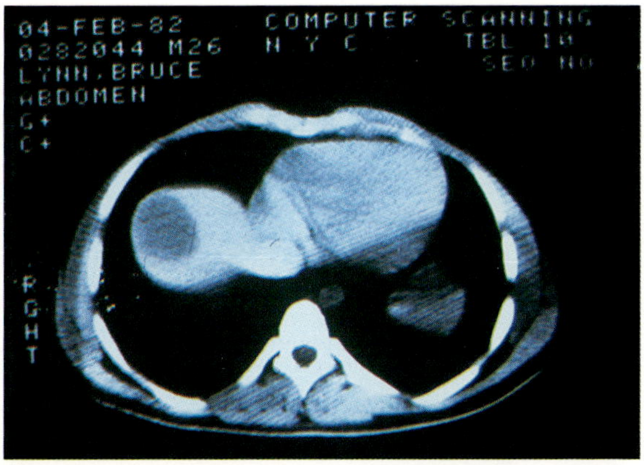
04-FEB-82
0282044 M26
LYNN,BRUCE
ABDOMEN
COMPUTER SCANNING
N Y C
TBL 10

A

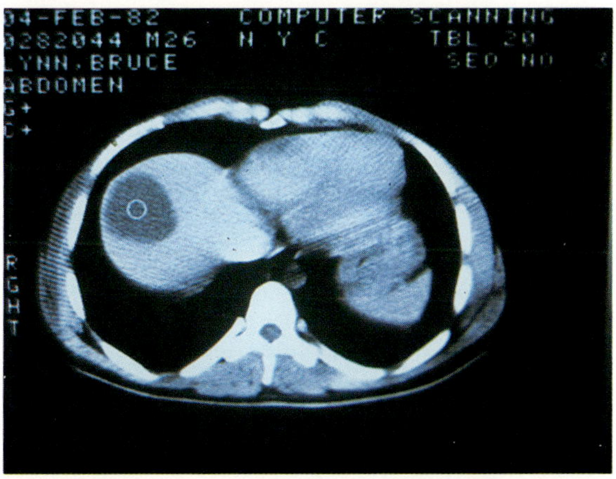
COMPUTER SCANNING
N Y C
TBL 20
LYNN,BRUCE

B

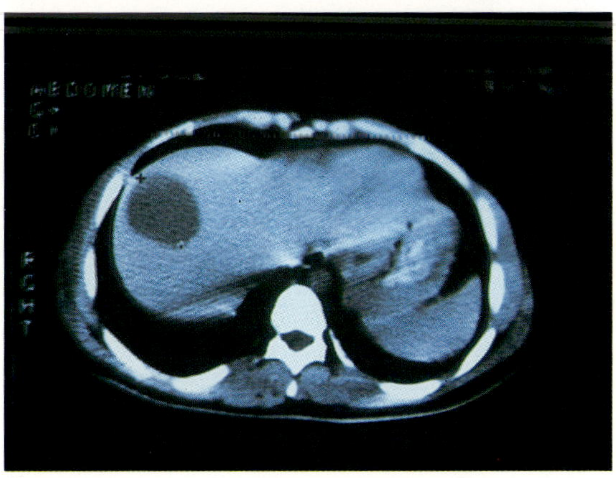

C

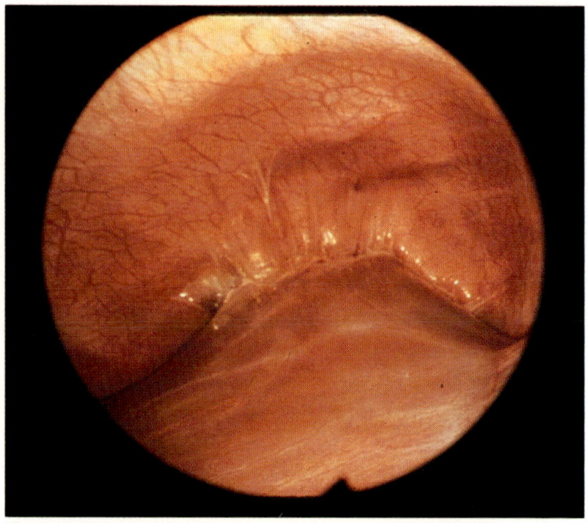

D

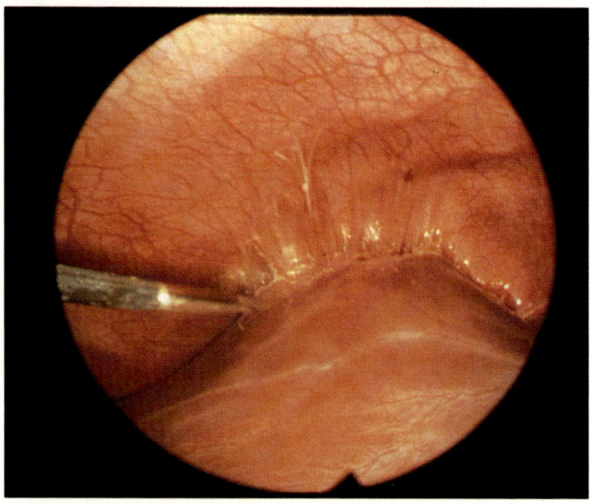

E

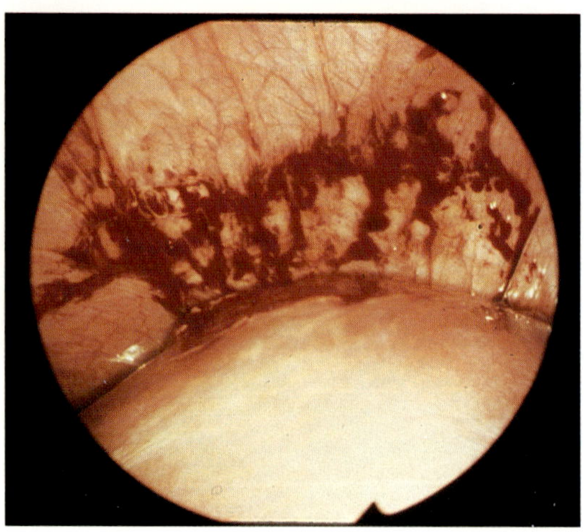

F

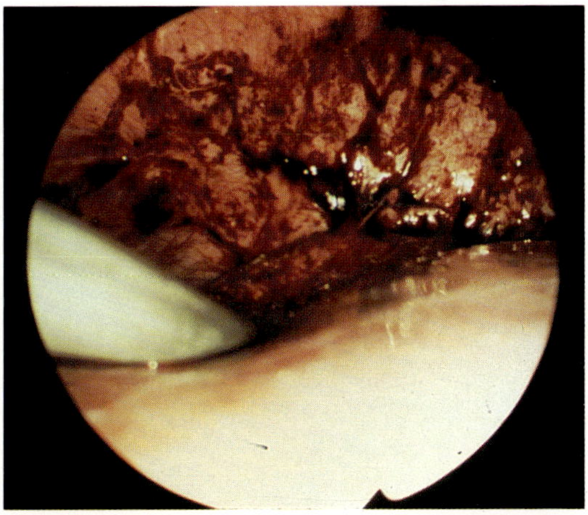

G

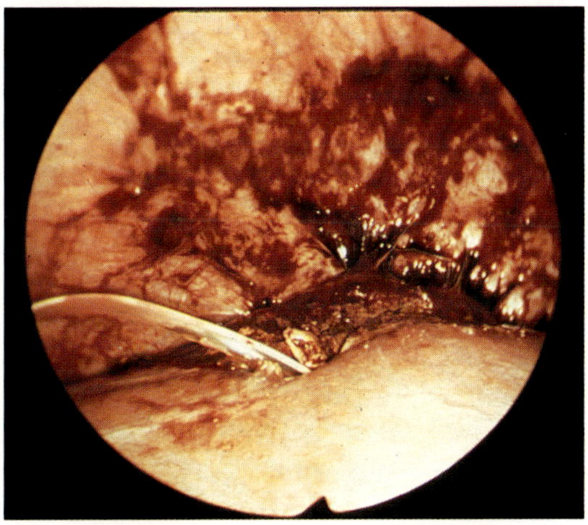

H

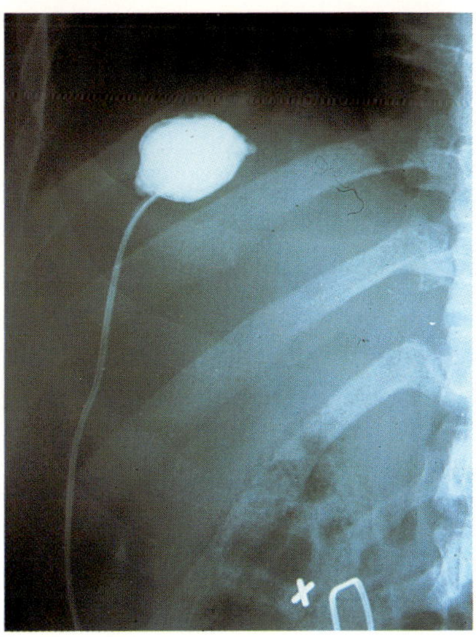

I

Case 6.2*A–L*

A 54-year-old female came to her gastroenterologist complaining of symptoms of increasing esophageal reflux. An upper gastrointestinal barium study revealed free reflux and extrinsic pressure on the greater curvature of the stomach. CT scan (Fig. 6.2**A** and Fig. 6.2**B**) revealed a large splenic cyst compressing the stomach. Figure 6.2**C** demonstrates the in situ appearance of the splenic cyst. The left hemidiaphragm is in the *background* with the phrenic vessels clearly seen. The normal phrenocolic ligament is present on the *far right.* Figure 6.2**D** views the aspirating needle poised to puncture the cyst. The phrenocolic ligament again is seen to the *right* of the needle. An avascular area on the surface of the cyst is easily identified. Figure 6.2**E** shows the needle in place with the cyst completely deflated. Three hundred cc of serous fluid was aspirated. Normal splenic tissue is now clearly visible in Figure 6.2**F**. A grasping forceps was inserted through the second puncture site, and it is lifting the decompressed cyst away from the surrounding structures as seen in Figure 6.2**G**. Figure 6.2**H** shows the scissors-coagulator beginning to cut a window in the wall of the cyst. Electrocautery was used to seal any blood vessels on the wall of the cyst before cutting with the scissors. The tip of the grasping forceps is visible at the *far right.* The scissors was inserted through a third puncture site. Figure 6.2**I** is a closeup view of the cyst window. The interior of the cyst is just visible beneath the scissors. Figure 6.2**J** is a view inside the cyst showing the typical trabeculated appearance of a benign cyst. The CT scan 2 months post-laparoscopy (Fig. 6.2**K**) shows a small residual cyst, and the CT scan 9 months later (Fig. 6.2**L**) reveals only a small defect in the spleen without evidence of recurrence. The usual treatment of a symptomatic splenic cyst is partial splenectomy whenever possible. However, it is a technically demanding operation with the distinct possibility of the need for a total splenectomy. Percutaneous aspiration under CT guidance is well-documented, but recurrence is common. The basis for opening a cyst-peritoneum window emanates from the similar treatment of a clear symptomatic liver cyst, in which drainage into the peritoneal cavity is an accepted modality. The peritoneal surface can reabsorb small amounts of serous fluid without difficulty. This procedure was performed under general anesthesia, and a setup for laparotomy was on standby in case bleeding occurred. The postlaparoscopy recovery was dramatic. Only minimal discomfort occurred, and the hospital stay was 4 days. The esophageal reflux abated immediately, and the patient has remained asymptomatic 4 years post procedure.

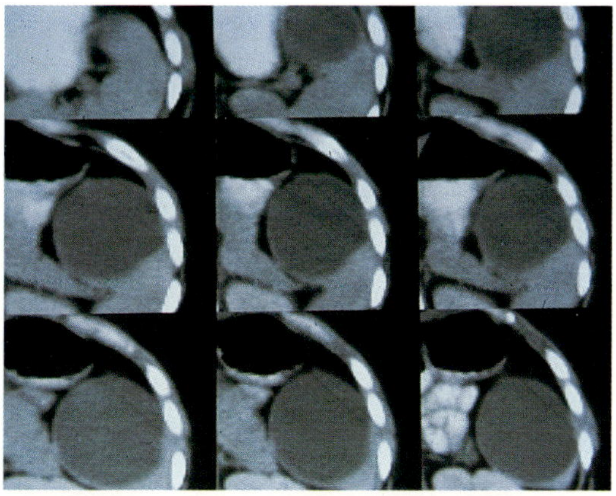

A

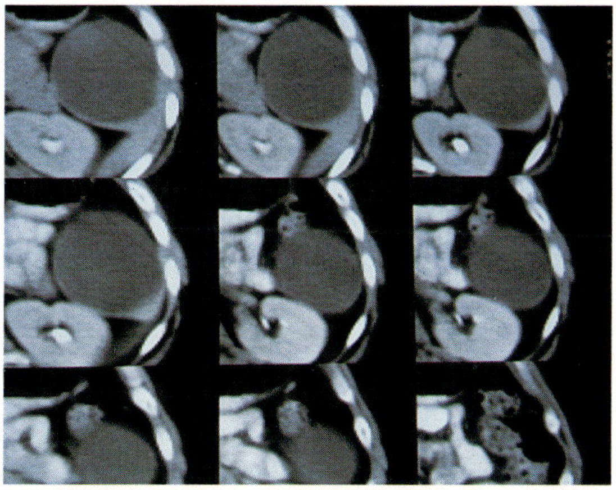

B

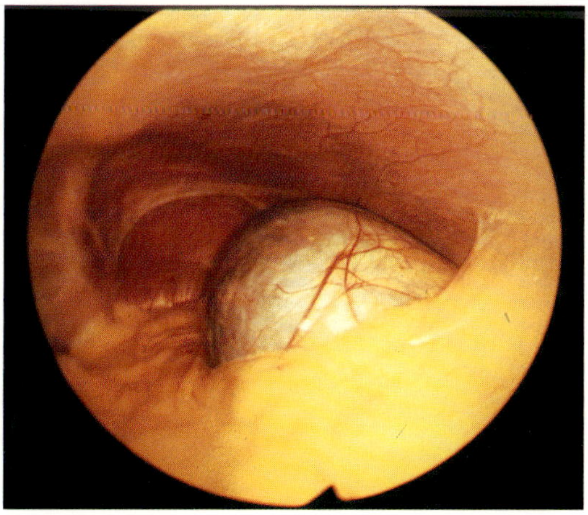

C

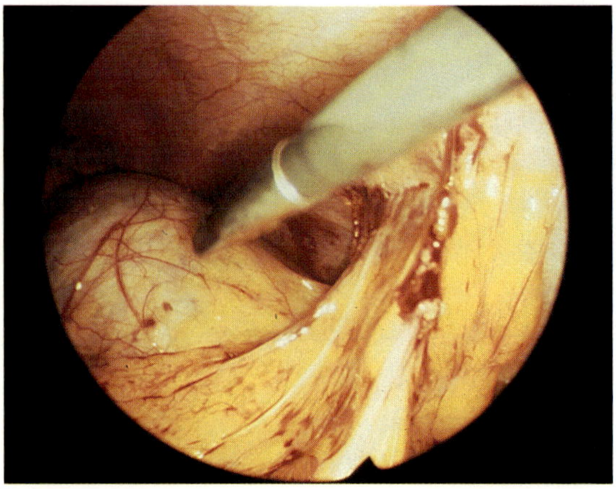

D

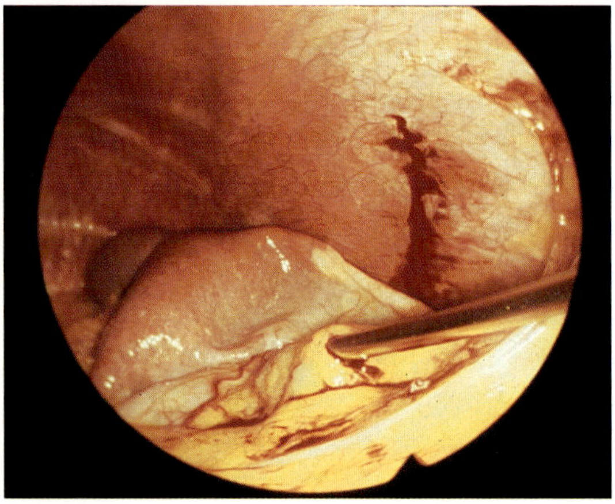

E

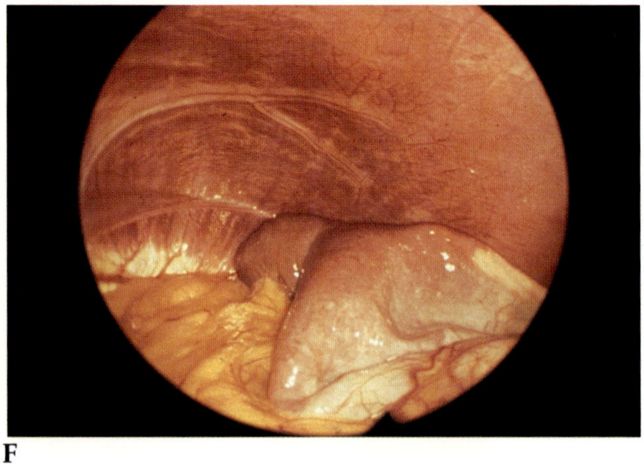

F

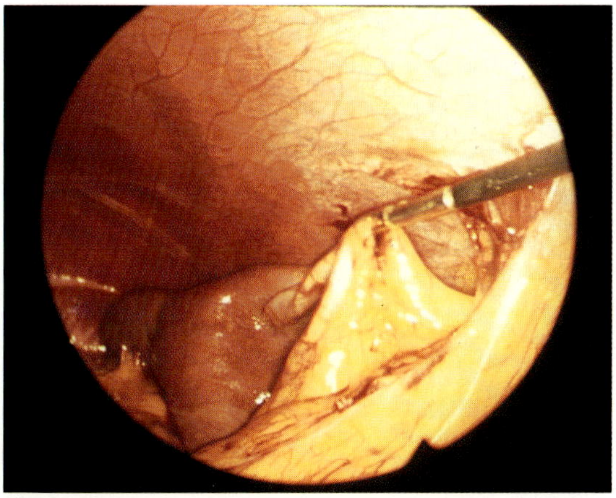

G

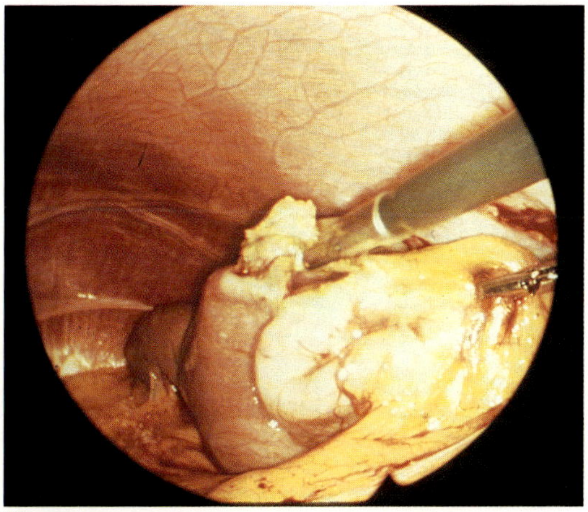

H

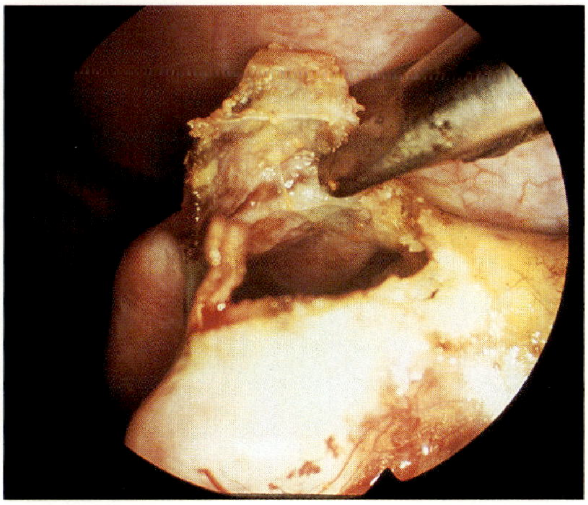

I

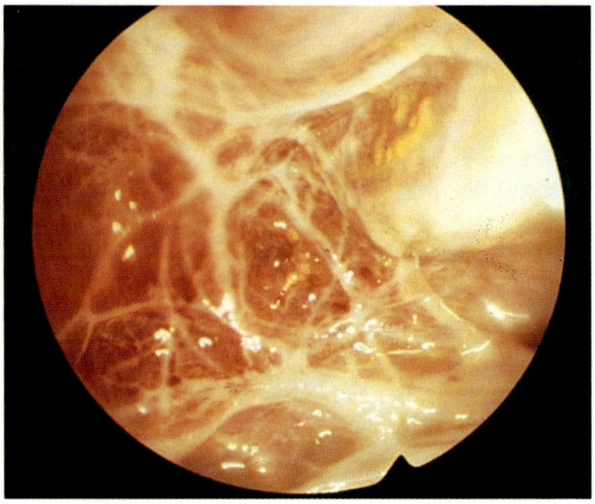
J

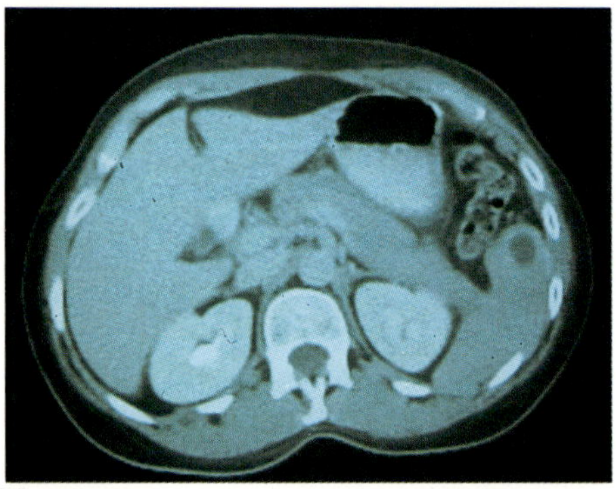
K

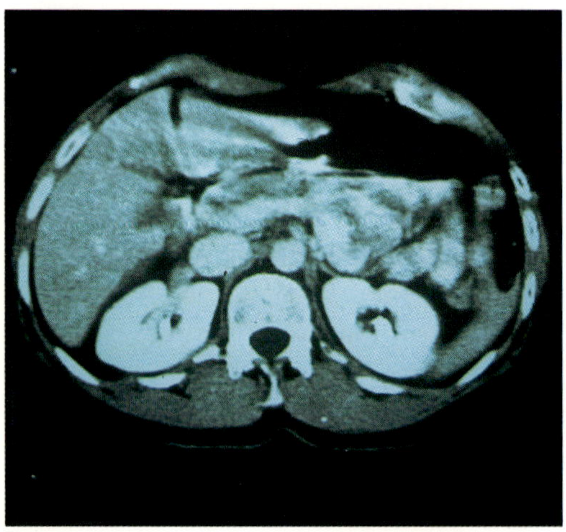
L

Case 6.3*A–D*

A 26-year-old male presented with multiple episodes of right lower quadrant pain. Several complete gastrointestinal workups were negative except for a nonfilled appendix. Figure 6.3**A** is a view of the right lower quadrant showing the appendix narrowed at its base and slight dilatation in its mid portion. There is no active inflammatory process present. A 5-mm second puncture sleeve and palpating probe are seen. There are several well-formed adhesions fixing the omentum to the right lateral abdominal wall that are indicative of some previous inflammatory process. The tip of the appendix is held with the Olympus bipolar grasping forceps (ordinarily used for laparoscopic tubal ligations). A hemostat is used to widen the tract around the second puncture sleeve. The pneumoperitoneum is then released through the trumpet valve on the laparoscope sleeve. This allows the cecum to reach the parietal peritoneal surface. If there are adhesions fixing the appendix, these should be lysed beforehand. The appendix is then extracted through the 5-mm second puncture incision, as seen in Figure 6.3**B**. The umbilicus and laparoscope sleeve are visible at the *far right*. The mesoappendix and base of the appendix are ligated on the abdominal wall (Fig. 6.3**C**). The base of the appendix is then pushed back into the abdomen, and the pneumoperitoeum is reexpanded. The appendiceal stump and mesoappendix are visually inspected with the laparoscope to ensure the security of the ligatures (Fig. 6.3**D**). Pathological diagnosis was a fibrotic appendix.

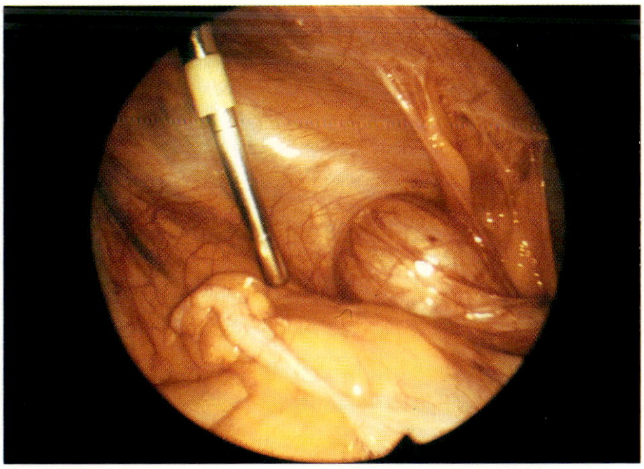

A

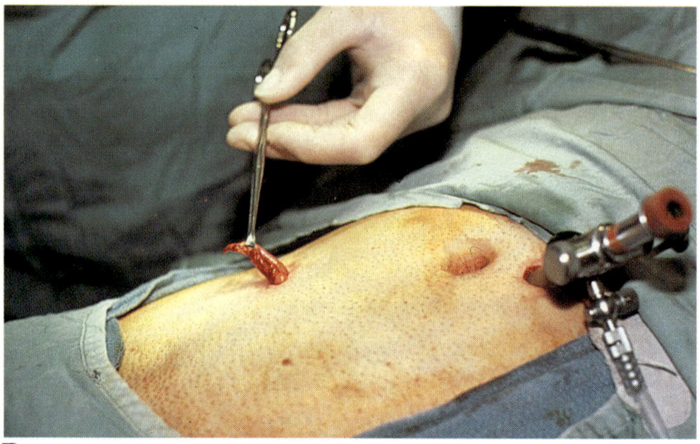

B

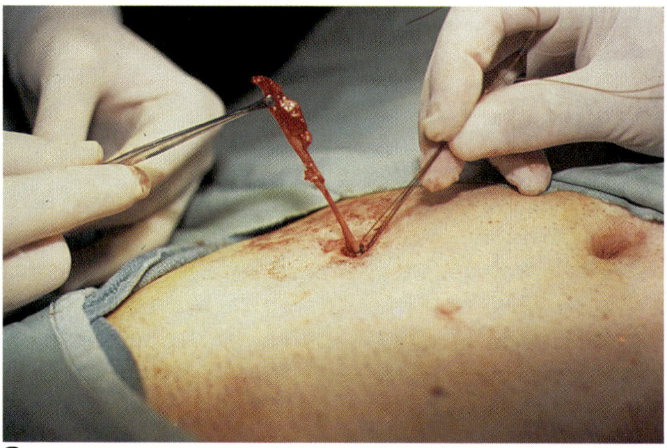

C

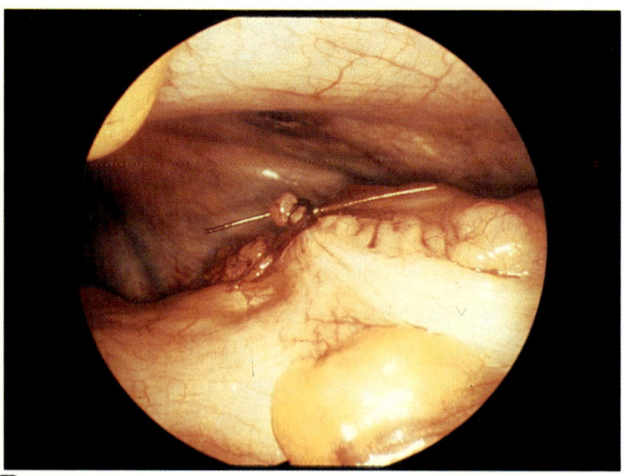

D

Case 6.4*A–C*

A 16-year-old male presented with multiple episodes of right lower quadrant pain over a 6-month period. On several occasions there was fever but no increase in the WBC count. Extensive evaluation of the gastrointestinal tract was negative. Figure 6.4**A** demonstrates a swollen appendix with hyperemia of its serosa. The serosa of the cecum is normal for comparison. The mesoappendix is slightly thickened. The tip of the appendix is secured by the Olympus bipolar forceps. The tract around the 5-mm second puncture site was widened as explained in Case 6.3. Figure 6.4**B** shows the appendix from the parietal surface pulled up through the second puncture tract. The base of the appendix and the cecum are clearly visible. After the appendix and mesoappendix were ligated and divided, the appendix was pushed back into the abdomen with the appendiceal ties still in place. Figure 6.4**C** shows this well. It is a safety measure in case bleeding from the appendiceal artery is identified. This will allow the area to be extracted back on the abdominal wall. The sutures are cut after laparoscopic visualization is complete. Pathological Dx: Mild appendiceal inflammation with lymphoid hyperplasia. Laparoscopic appendectomy is a well-accepted procedure in several European centers. Its major use is in cases of chronic right lower quadrant pain syndromes, in which visualization of the appendix at the time of laparoscopy demonstrates appendiceal pathology. The procedure is performed under general anesthesia, and standby instruments for laparotomy should be in place. In the author's experience, the patients have much less abdominal discomfort and ileus because of the small incisions and because there is virtually no handling of the intestine. Usual in-hospital time is 2 days.

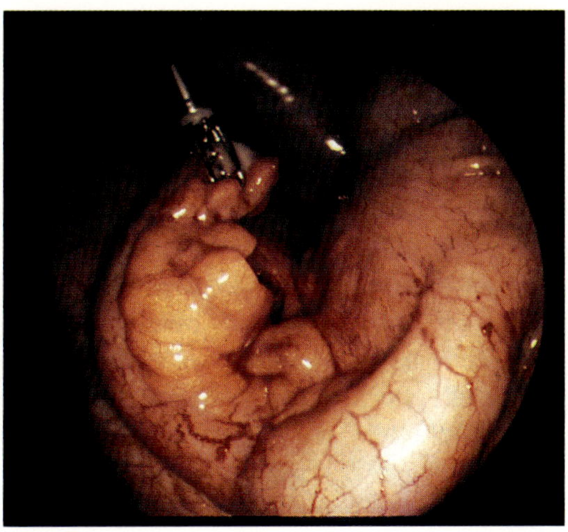

A

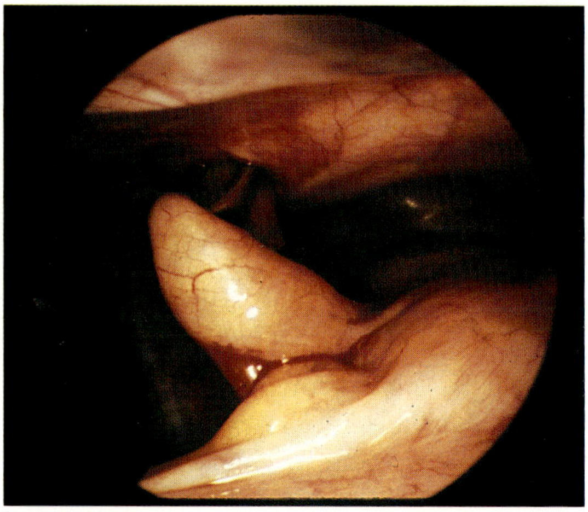

B

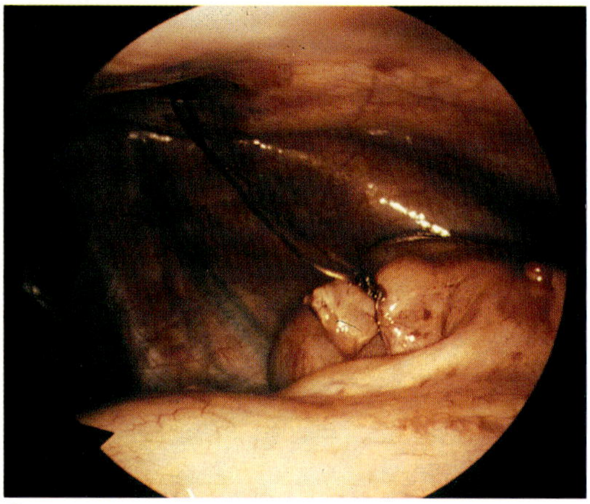

C

Case 6.5*A–C*

A 26-year-old female 5 years status post-appendectomy presented with recurrent right lower quadrant pain just lateral to a standard McBurney incision. The pain began soon after the appendectomy and never varied in its position. Multiple gastrointestinal workups were negative. This patient already has been presented as Case 2-30. Figure 6.5**A** shows the in situ appearance of the right lower quadrant. The cecum is free of adhesions while the ascending colon adheres to the right lateral abdominal wall directly under the previous incision. The second puncture sleeve is positioned by the cecum. As the laparoscopy was performed under local anesthesia, the patient was able to state that the pain was reproduced exactly when the adhesions were pulled by the palpating probe. Figure 6.5**B** reveals the scissors properly positioned to sever the adhesions. Note the clear area between the bowel wall and the abdominal wall. Figure 6.5**C** demonstrates the complete lysis, and the colon back in its normal position. The omentum was manipulated to overlay the ascending colon.

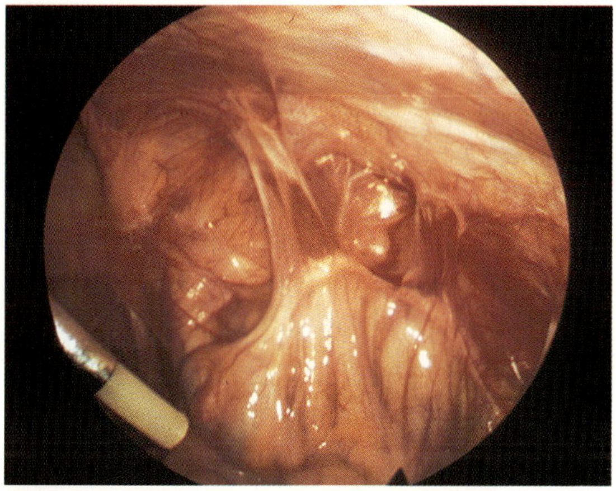

A

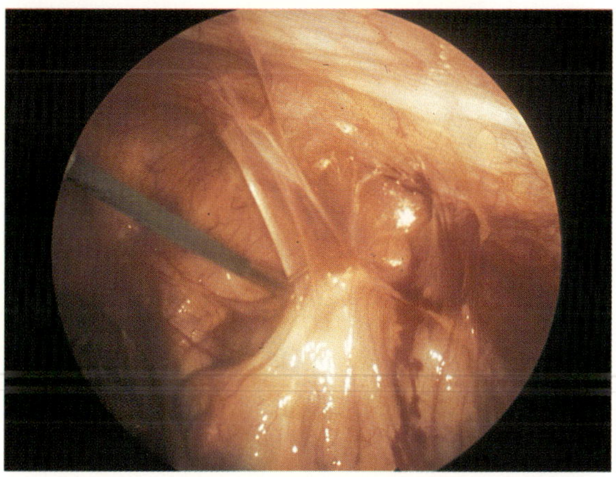

B

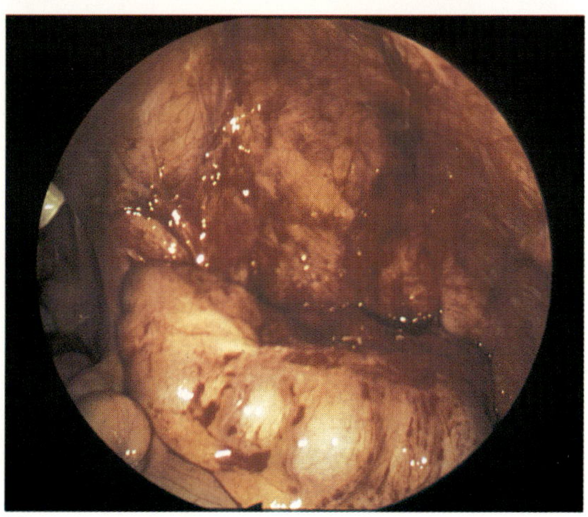

C

Case 6.6*A–C*

A 30-year-old female complained of recurrent right upper quadrant pain for 3 years following an appendectomy. Complete gastrointestinal workup was negative. Figure 6.6**A** demonstrates the in situ appearance. Note the two single-band adhesions between the ascending colon and the parietal peritoneum. Manipulation of both mimicked the pain. Figure 6.6**B** shows the laparoscopic scissors in place away from the bowel and parietal peritoneum. The small blood vessels in the adhesions do not require electrocauterization. Figure 6.6**C** shows the colon back in its normal position. A small amount of blood is present near the hepatic flexure. As stated in the chapter on abdominal pain, an awake patient is important so that he/she can help localize the adhesion or adhesions causing the pain. The extensive lysis of adhesions, as in Case 6.5, re-

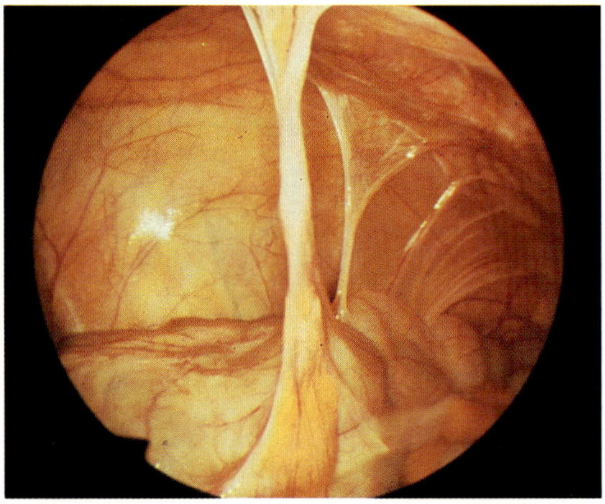

A

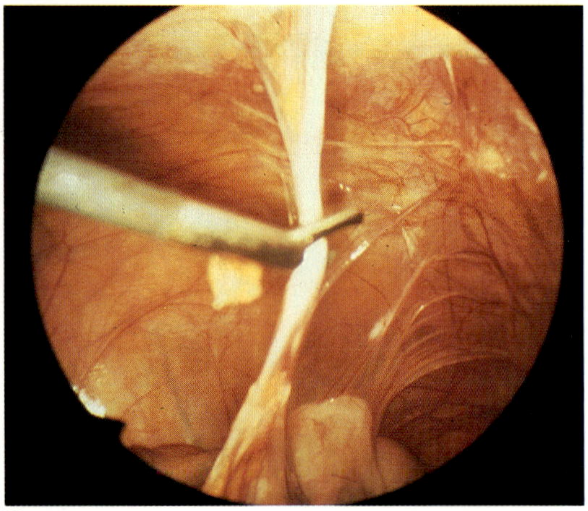

B

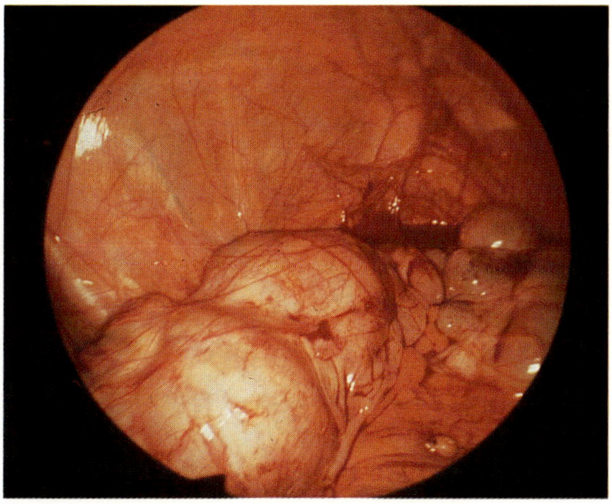

C

quired only mild intravenous sedation during the procedure. Care must be taken by the laparoscopist to avoid pulling on the parietal peritoneum to ensure the comfort of the patient. Occasionally, the adhesions can be vascularized, in which case the application of electrocautery will be necessary before dividing the adhesion.

Case 6.7*A–C*

A 50-year-old female on chronic ambulatory peritoneal dialysis (CAPD) for 3 years presented with sudden bleeding from the Tenckhoff® catheter and inability to flush the catheter. The abdominal examination was benign. Complete coagulation workup was normal. Figure 6.7**A** demonstrates the in situ appearance of the previously placed peritoneal dialysis catheter occluded with fibrin blood clot. The catheter enters the abdomen at the 11 o'clock position and enters the pelvis in the 4 o'clock position. A 3-mm second puncture sleeve penetrating the abdominal wall is visible behind the dialysis catheter. Figure 6.7**B** reveals the length of clot extending down the catheter tubing. The second puncture sleeve is again visible behind the catheter. Part of the dialysis catheter is also clearly seen. A 3-mm grasping forceps was inserted through the second puncture sleeve, and the blood clot was removed from the dialysis tubing. Figure 6.7**C** shows the clot being extracted from the abdominal cavity through the 3-mm second puncture tract. A clear dialysis catheter is now seen just above the pointer. Laparoscopic manipulations of intraabdominal catheters is straightforward if adhesions do not preclude its visualization. CAPD catheters not infrequently malfunction secondary to fibrin deposition or omental adhesions. The laparoscopic unblocking of these catheters will often allow their continued use. As peritoneal dialysis requires an intact abdominal wall, it is important to use a small laparoscope for these therapeutic manipulations. In this case, a 5-mm laparoscope was chosen. After its removal, the fascial defect requires a water-tight sutured closure. Local anesthesia was used throughout this procedure.

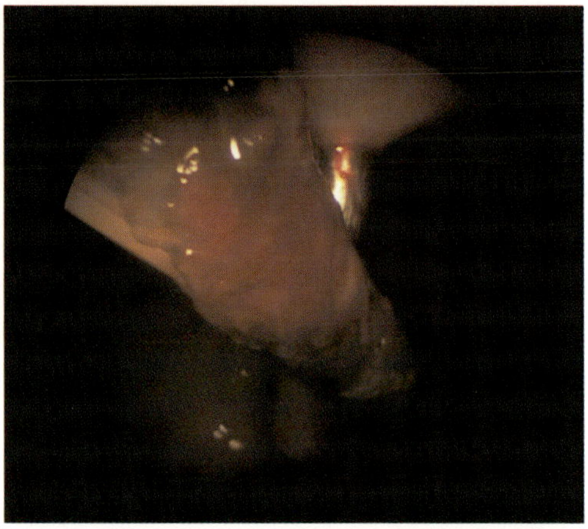

A

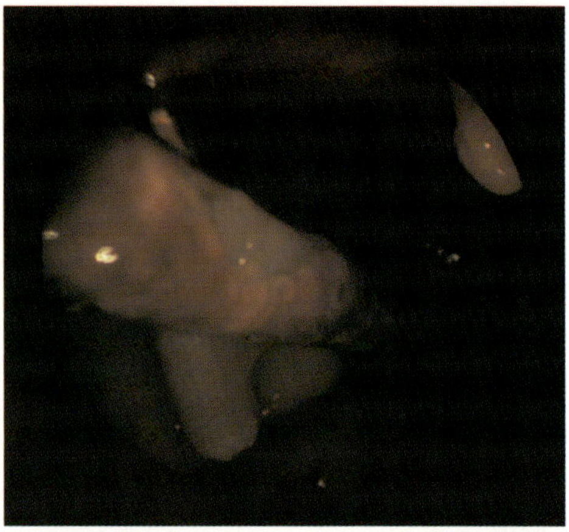

B

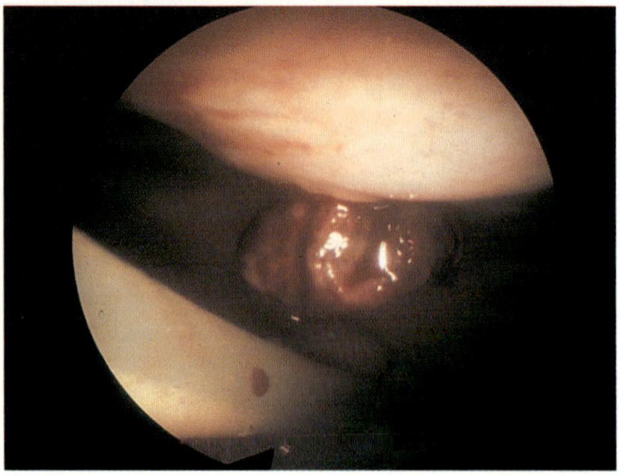

C

Case 6.8*A–H*

A 68-year-old female with chronic renal failure needed placement of a Tenckhoff® dialysis catheter for CAPD. Figure 6.8**A** shows a 3-cm incision placed slightly below and to the *left* of the umbilicus. Two army-navy retractors are seen. A pneumoperitoneum is introduced with the Veress needle in a standard fashion. Figure 6.8**B** demonstrates the 5-mm laparoscopic sleeve in place. The umbilicus is seen just superior to the sleeve. Figure 6.8**C** reveals the in situ appearance of lower abdomen with the parietal peritoneum and the omentum clearly seen. The laparoscope is removed after visualization of a clear pelvis. A purse string suture of chromic is placed in the anterior fascia close to the laparoscopic sleeve (Fig. 6.8**D**). It is left untied. The sleeve is removed, and the Tenckhoff® catheter is inserted into the pelvic area through the 5-mm puncture produced by the laparoscopic trocar insertion. This maneuver is greatly facilitated by using a metal introducer inside the Tenckhoff® catheter. Figure 6.8**E** shows the catheter entering the abdomen and the untied purse string suture. The umbilicus is above and to the left of the incision. The catheter is advanced until the distal Dacron cuff is just above the anterior fascia (Fig. 6.8**F**). The cuff is grasped with a forceps and placed below the anterior fascia. The purse string suture is now tied (Fig. 6.8**G**). The catheter is then tunneled out in the standard surgical manner, leaving the proximal Dacron cuff at least 2 cm deep from the exit site to the subcutaneous tissue. The incision is then closed with a subcuticular suture (Fig. 6.8**H**). There are several advantages to placing a Tenckhoff® catheter with the aid of the laparoscope. The incision necessary is rarely larger than 3 cm. General anesthesia has never been necessary. The pelvis is inspected visually and, therefore, proper placement of the catheter is ensured. If any adhesions are found, they may be lysed laparoscopically. No retraction of the parietal peritoneum is necessary, thereby causing almost no discomfort during the procedure. The operating time is rarely more than 20 min.

There are some technical considerations that merit comment. The outer diameter of the Tenckhoff® catheter is 4.9 mm. Therefore, the 5-mm laparoscope and sleeve should be used to puncture the abdominal wall. The laparoscopic puncture should be through the same hole as the Veress needle puncture, as a water-tight seal is necessary. The author's preference is the precurled Tenckhoff® catheter. The metal stylet introducer greatly eases the placement of the catheter into its proper position. The author strongly suggests its use. This technique of placement also allows immediate use if acute dialysis is necessary.

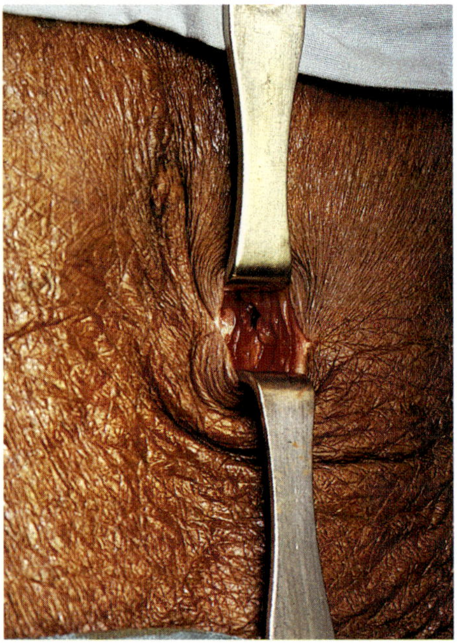

A

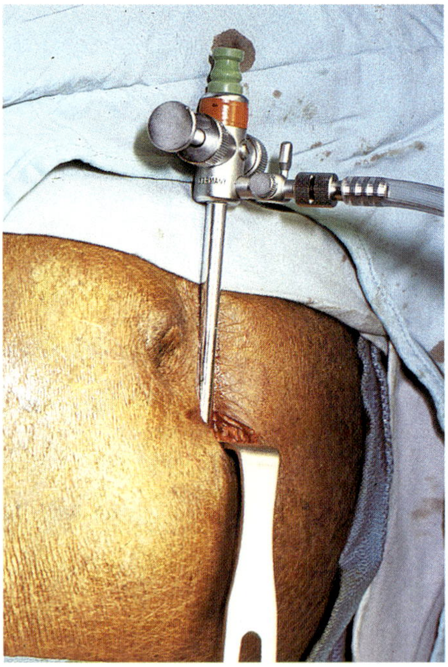

B

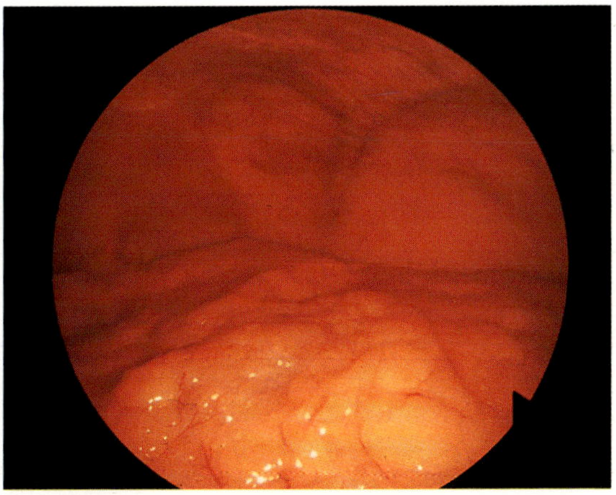

C

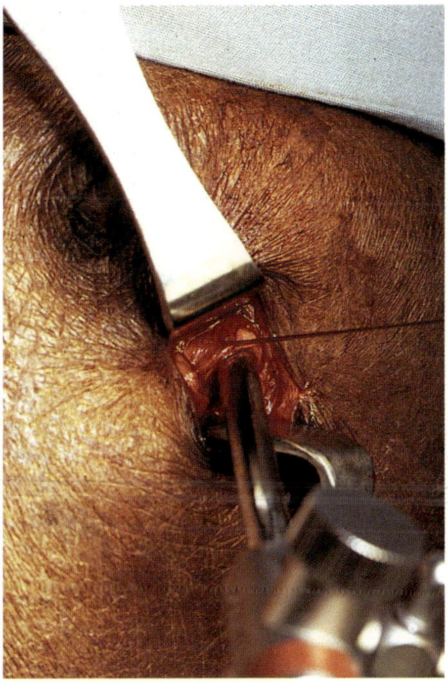

D

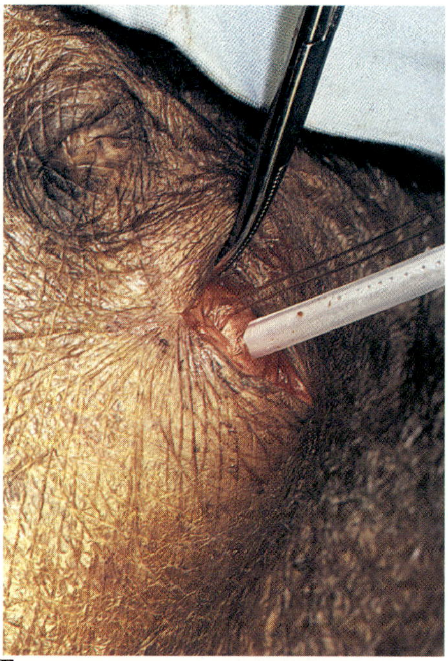

E

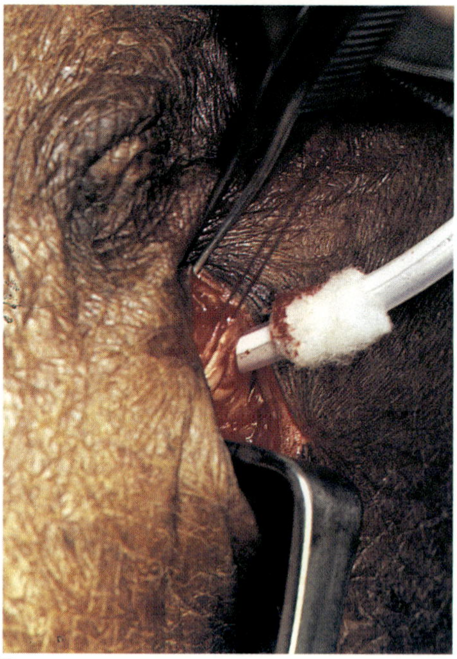

F

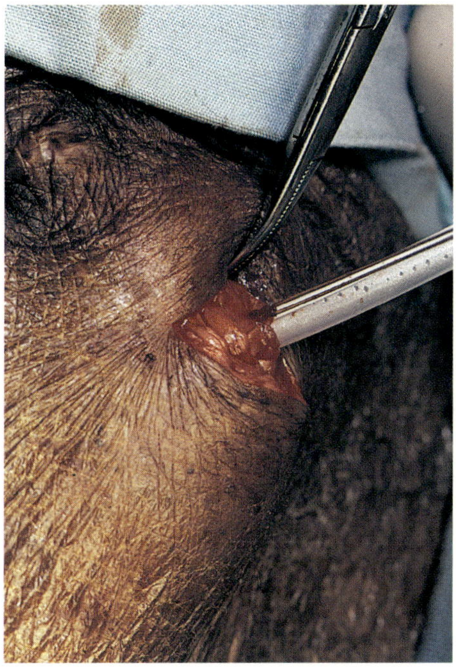

G

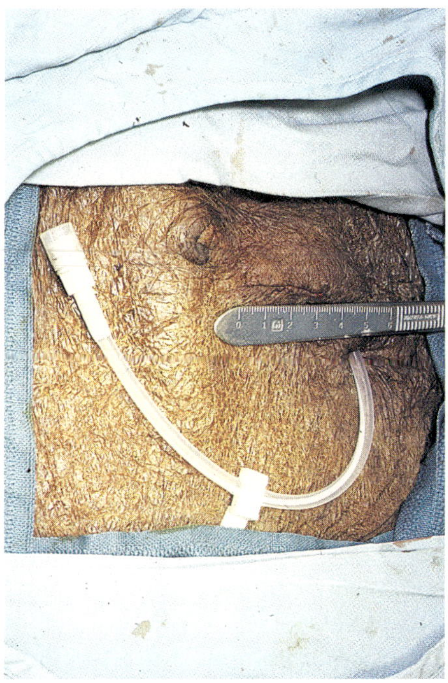

H

LAPAROSCOPIC CHOLECYSTECTOMY

Case 6.9*A–P*

A 26-year-old female with multiple episodes of biliary colic. Sonographic examination of the right-upper quadrant revealed multiple stones in a non-thickened gall bladder. The common bile duct measured 4mms and the pancreas was normal. An oral cholecystogram revealed a functional gall bladder with seven stones totaling greater than 3 cm., thereby excluding extracorporeal shock wave lithotripsy (ESWL). Cholecystectomy was recommended which was accomplished by laparoscopic technique.

Figure 6.9**A** shows the four punctures in the abdominal wall which allow introduction of the necessary instrumentation to perform a cholecystectomy. The umbilical and left-sided sleeves are 10 mms each. The two portals under the right rib margin are 5 mms in diameter. The video camera (Olympus OTV-S2) is attached to the umbilical portal as seen in Figure 6.9**A**. The suction-irrigator is inserted through the medial-upper port, a grasping forceps is placed via the right lateral port, and the hook-electrode (crochet) is directed through the left lateral port. The insitu appearance of the gall bladder, cystic duct, common hepatic duct, common bile duct, and cystic artery are clearly seen in Figure 6.9**B**. A grasping forceps is applied to the gall bladder neck (not visible in Figure 6.9**B**), and traction is placed laterally and superiorly to splay open the biliary structures (Fig. 6.9**B**). Figure 6.9**C** demonstrates the completed dissection of the cystic duct. The cystic artery is being dissected with the 5 mm hook-electrode, which is inserted through the left side portal. A 5 mm reducing sleeve must be placed into the 10 mm opening to accept the smaller instrument. The neck of the gall bladder is to the left, and the liver is retracted upward with the 5 mm suction-irrigator. The completed dissection of the cystic artery and duct is seen in Figure 6.9**D**. The cystic duct and artery are secured by titanium clips as demonstrated in Figure 6.9**E**. The common bile duct is seen clearly to the right. Notice the double clip on the common duct side of the cystic artery. The endo clip-applicator (United States Surgical Corporation, Norwalk, Conn) and cartridge insert are shown in Figure 6.9**F**. Each cartridge contains 20 titanium clips which are fed into the jaws of the applicator by simply depressing a button at the top of the handle. Figure 6.9**G** demonstrates the clipped cystic duct just before its transection with the 5mm microscissors. The cystic duct-common bile duct junction is clearly seen at the bottom. The cystic artery is cut in like fashion. The gall bladder is then dissected from the liver bed in a retrograde manner using the hook-electrode as seen in Figure 6.9**H**. The gall bladder is grasped with a forceps and placed on top of the right lobe of the liver (Fig. 6.9**I**), so that inspection of the liver bed may proceed without obscuring the visual field. Figure 6.9**J** demonstrates the liver bed after the gall bladder has been completely dissected free from the liver. The titanium clip on the cystic duct stump is visible at the bottom right. Gentle upward traction by the suction-irrigator on the liver allows excellent visualization of the liver bed. The laparoscope and video camera are moved to the left abdominal portal, and a grasping forceps is inserted through the umbilical sleeve. The gall bladder is held at the cut portion of the cystic duct as shown in Figure 6.9**K**. Care must be taken not to dislodge the titanium clip from the cystic duct during this maneuver. The gall bladder is then pulled into the 10 mm umbilical sleeve, and the sleeve is withdrawn from the abdominal wall. The gall bladder is secured with hemostats on the abdominal wall at the umbilical incision site (Fig. 6.9**L**). The grasping forceps and 10 mm sleeve are seen. The upper abdomen is to the left. A small incision is made in the gall bladder to allow the bile to be aspirated with a small neuro suction. The gall bladder is seen visually, as it appears from the inside of the abdomen, at all times by the video camera (Figure 6.9**M**). There is still some bile in the gall bladder, which accounts for its globular shape. Figure 6.9**N** shows the gall bladder being removed from the abdomen through the umbilical incision. The laparoscope and video camera, which were inserted through the left abdominal portal previously are seen at the top of Figure 6.9**N**. Figure 6.9**O** shows the closed skin incisions immediately after the procedure, and Figure 6.9**P** illustrates the wounds ten days after the operation.

(*Discussion text follows on page 143*)

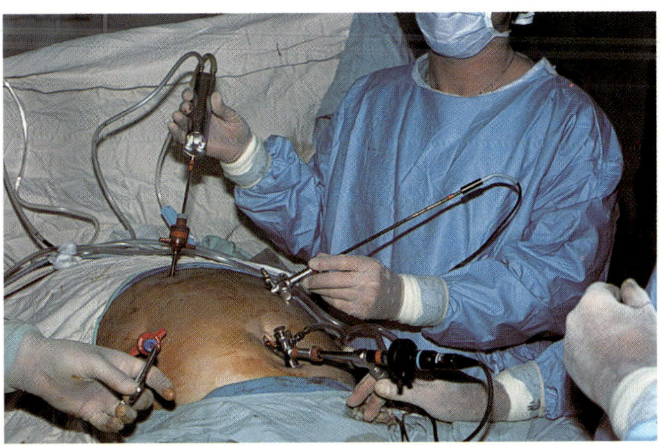

A

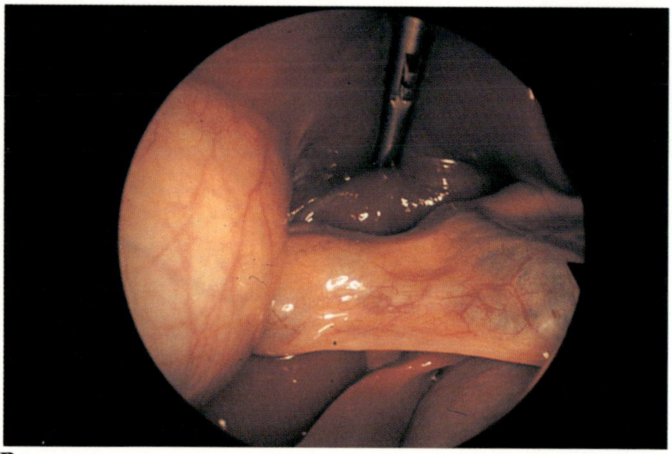

B

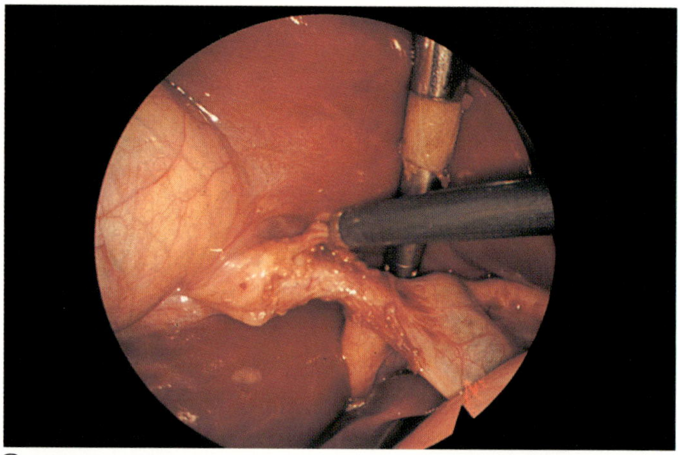

C

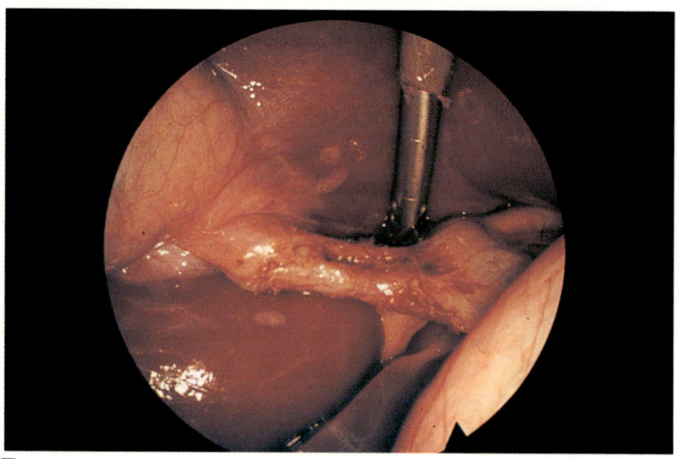

D

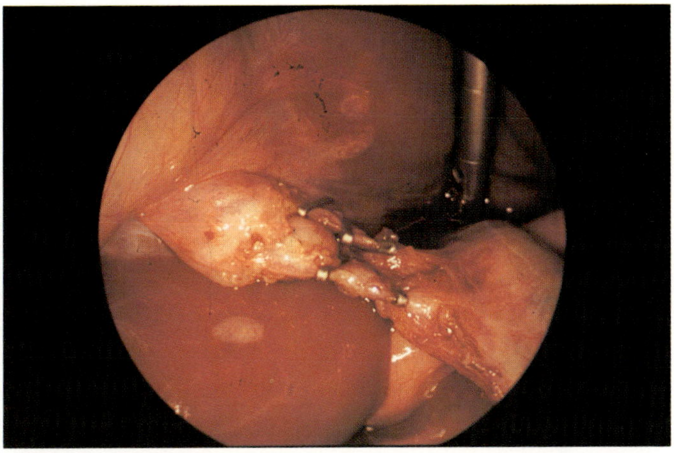

E

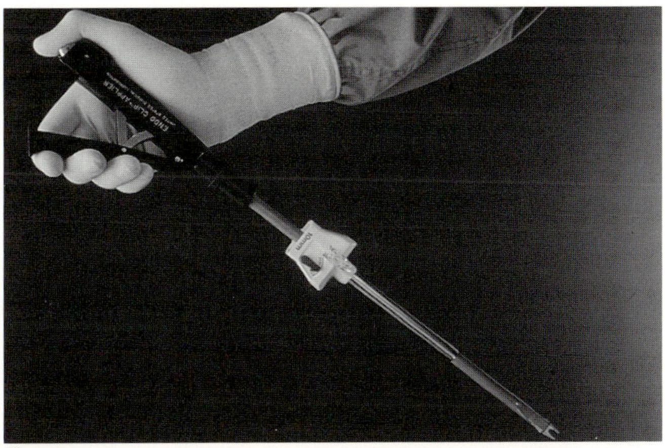

F

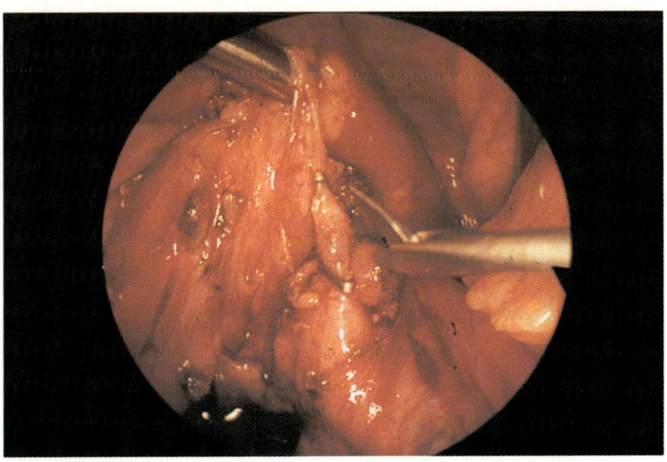

G

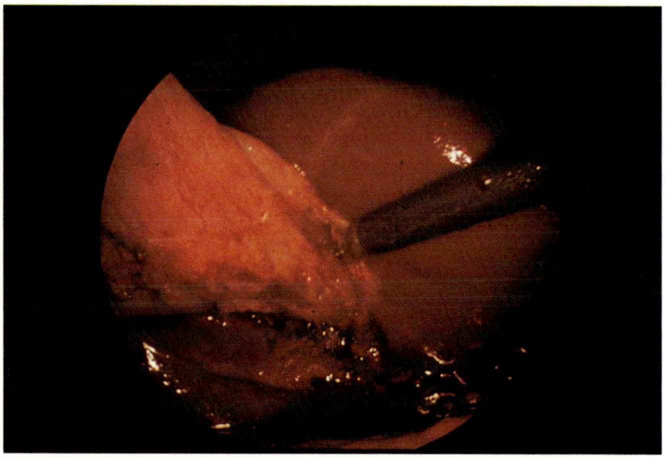

H

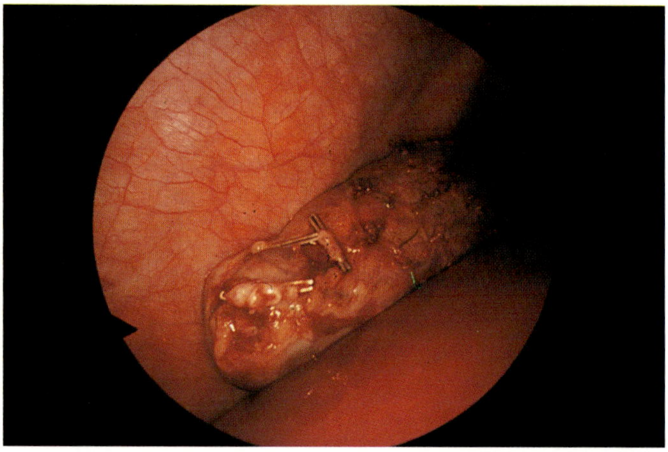

I

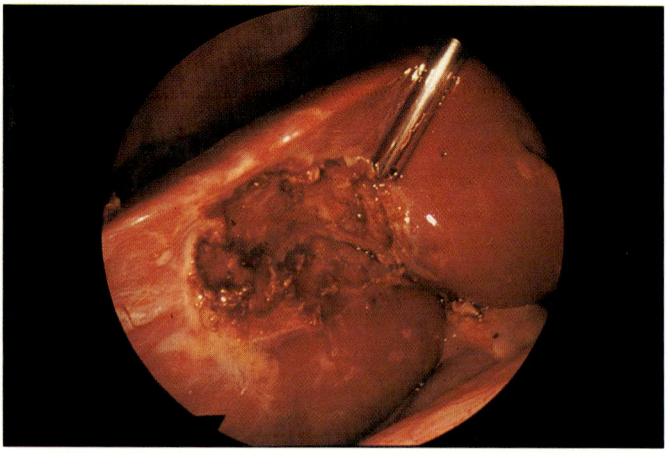

J

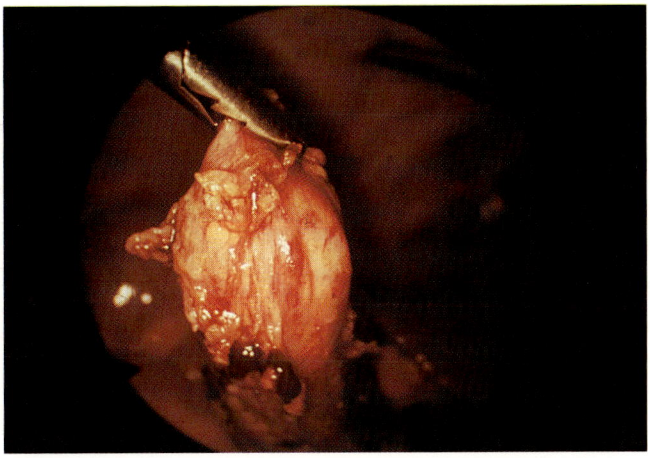

K

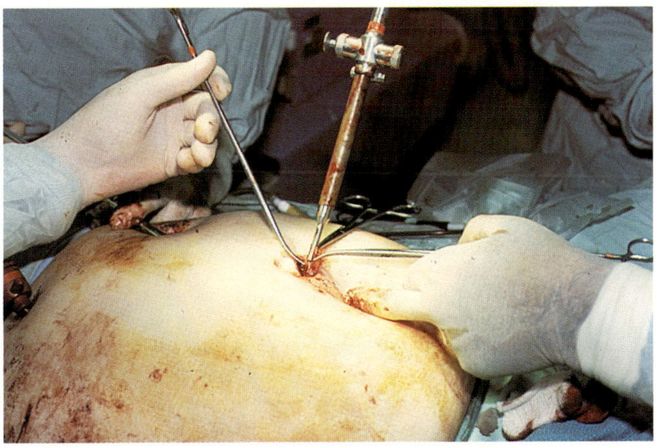

L

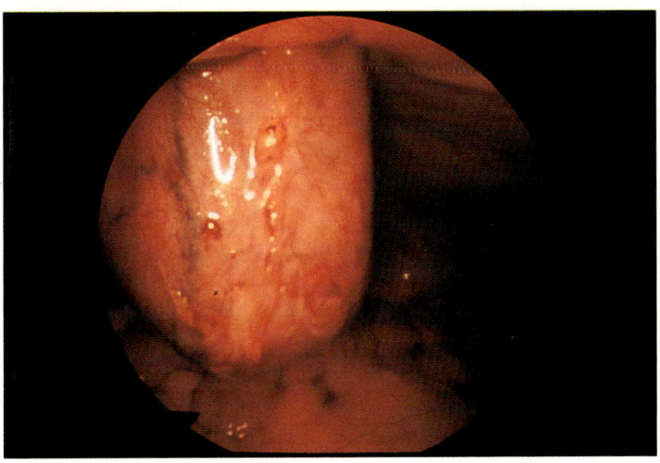

M

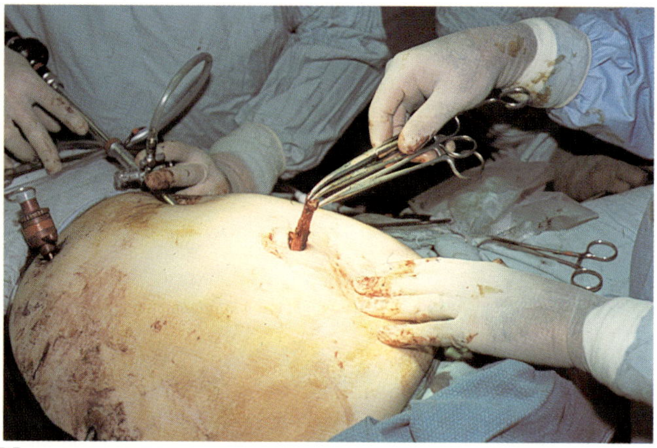

N

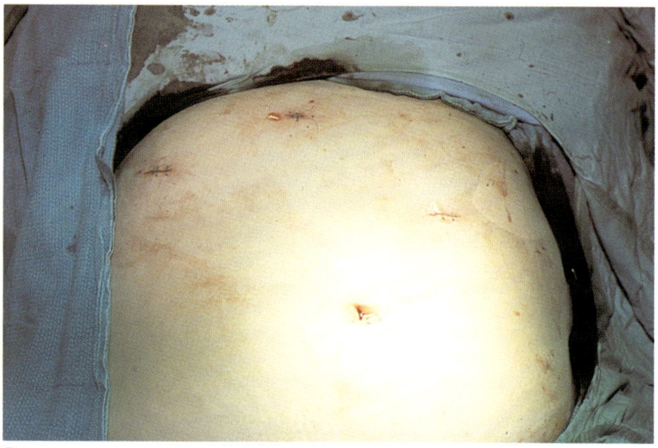

O

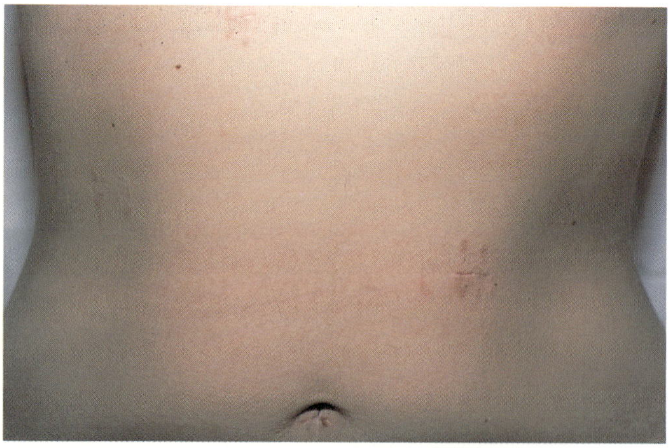

P

Discussion

Laparoscopic cholecystectomy will dramatically change the surgical and medical approach to significant numbers of patients with biliary tract disease. The early experience with this new modality is extremely encouraging. Its exact place in the armamentarium of the surgeon is only now being studied, however, previous operative laparoscopic experience should be mandatory before attempting this procedure.

The present indication for using laparoscopic cholecystectomy is symptomatic biliary colic. Acute cholecystitis is presently best approached by traditional open surgery, but that may change as further experience is gained with this new technique. Known choledocholithiasis in association with symptomatic cholelithiasis may be treated with preoperative endoscopic retrograde cholangiopancreatography (ERCP), followed by laparoscopic cholecystectomy. Of course, the standard open surgical procedure is also a viable option. Intraoperative (laparoscopic) cholangiography may be performed as well, and its use is to be encouraged. The use of preoperative intravenous cholangiography for evaluation of the common bile duct is used routinely in Europe. The author uses prophylactic antibiotics in both laparoscopic and traditional cholecystectomies. It is the author's hope that a multi-institutional trial be started by surgeons familiar with this technique, so that its proper place is defined for all surgeons.

A significant amount of new instrumentation is necessary to perform laparoscopic cholecystectomy. The video camera and color monitor are absolutely necessary, as this technique requires the coordination of two operators. The new six-liter-per-minute high insufflator is also necessary to keep an adequate pneumoperitoneum. These insufflators allow the surgeon to preset a maximum pressure that will not be exceeded; this gives an extra element of safety for the patient. The author uses the Olympus CLV-10 light source and the Olympus video camera. As significant electrocautery is used during the procedure, CO_2 should be the insufflating gas of choice for this procedure. A variety of grasping forceps and scissors are needed and are available from various suppliers. The dissection of the cystic artery, cystic duct and gall bladder fossa is performed with the hook electrode. The endo clip-applicator has simplified and shortened the technique; it is recommended that the endo clip-applicator rather than the single use applicator be used. The suction-irrigator is necessary for the same reasons as in traditional surgery.

The advantages of laparoscopic cholecystectomy to the patient are dramatic: (1) The post operative pain is significantly less; (2) As there is no manipulation of the bowel, post operative ileus is distinctly uncommon; (3) Most patients are fed the night of surgery; (4) The average length of the hospital stay is two days, and the average time before returning to work is one week post procedure.

There will, of course, be occasions in which patients will need to be converted to open cholecystectomy. For this reason, informed consent must be taken beforehand.

7

EMERGENCY LAPAROSCOPY

George Berci

Root and his co-workers introduced abdominal lavage for detection of intraabdominal bleeding.[1] At a later stage, it was found that surgical exploration was not required in every case of hemoperitoneum and that the incidence of unnecessary diagnostic laparotomy in cases of blunt abdominal trauma is about 20%.[2] In one-fifth of patients, no visceral injury or significant bleeding site was found and, therefore, no further intervention was necessary. Even with the introduction of computer tomography (CT), a complex and expensive diagnostic study has not eliminated unnecessary laparotomies.[3] Patients who were explored and for whom no surgical treatment was required represented a significant morbidity and expense for patients with extended hospitalization.

The concept of laparoscopic examination of intraabdominal organs on an emergency basis was introduced by several authors, including this author.[4, 5] We developed a miniature laparoscope that is almost identical to the lavage catheter. Small instruments are easier, faster, and safer to introduce than large or standard instruments. Emergency laparoscopy can be performed in the ER on a stretcher or in the Intensive Care Unit at the bedside of the patient. The procedure is performed under local anesthesia with IV sedation. The patient's condition must be monitored continuously throughout the examination.

INDICATIONS

The indications for emergency laparoscopy are as follows: (*a*) mental obtundation; (*b*) history or evidence of blunt abdominal trauma or abdominal stab wounds; (*c*) unexplained hypotension; (*d*) equivocal signs of abdominal examination.

There are many conditions in which intraabdominal conditions are difficult to discover due to the patient's mental condition (head trauma, alcoholism, drug ingestion, multiple injuries, etc.). Hypotension can have many possible causes, if during the evaluation, the etiology is not evident, intraabdominal hemorrhage or other acute events will be included in the differential diagnosis. In the early phase of hemorrhage or perforations, the usual signs of an intraabdominal catastrophy can be absent. There are many clinical situations in which a rapid and accurate diagnosis with proper assessment of treatment priorities can influence the eventual outcome for patients who have sustained a severe trauma.

Peritoneal lavage is an overly sensitive examination. There are in fact several overlaps between positive and negative results so that interpretation frequently remains in doubt in a difficult clinical situation for which the test is intended.

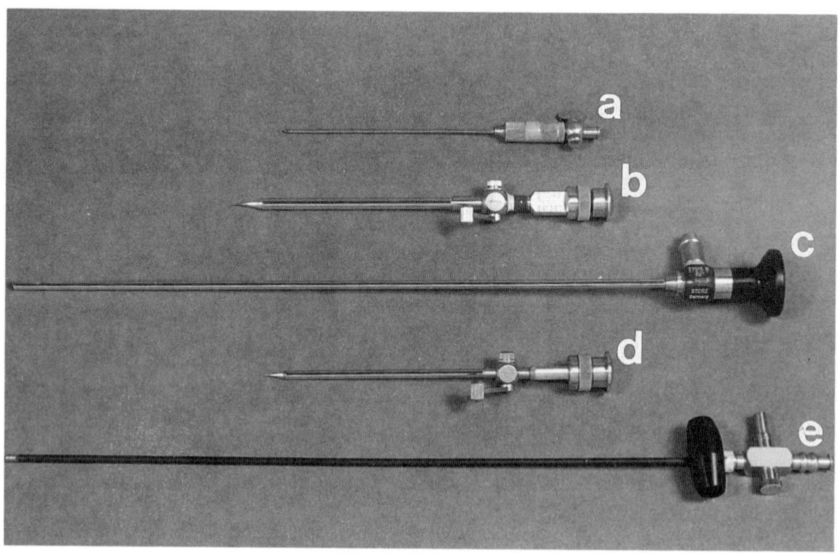

Figure 7.1
The minilaparoscopy set. (**A**) Pneumoperitoneum needle; (**B**) 5-mm trocar with stylet; (**C**) 30° foroblique telescope with fiber light guide incorporated (OD, 4.1 mm); (**D**) 5-mm accessory trocar; (**E**) Suction-coagulation-palpation probe.

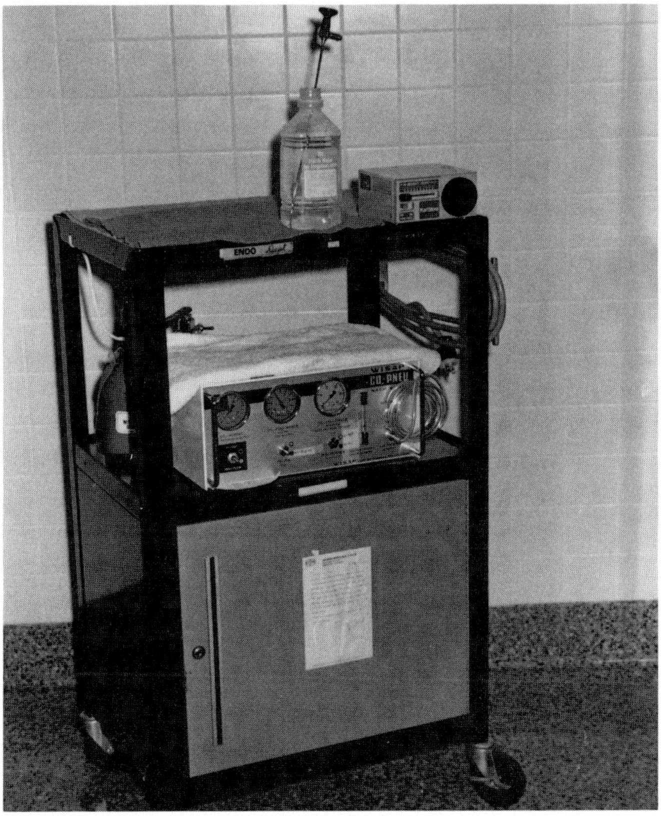

Figure 7.2.
Mobile cart in which the instruments, gowns, etc. are kept sterile and locked. It can be wheeled around (Emergency Room, Intensive Care Unit, etc). **Top:** The sterile telescope is inserted in a preheated (microwave oven), sterile saline container. This process avoids fogging of the telescope. The light source is seen beside the telescope. **Middle:** Co_2 (N_2O) insufflator. The gas cylinders are mounted behind. **Bottom:** Storage compartment.

TECHNIQUE

A laparoscopic instrument is prepared on a mobile cart. This set includes a 4-mm telescope* with a 30° forward oblique view. A pneumoperitoneal needle, accessory trocar (4-mm) palpation probe, which acts as a suction coagulation, a probe with a trumpet valve for evacuation and electric contact for connection to an electrosurgical unit and the suction coagulation palpation probe are the most important accessories. It acts as an "extended finger" of the endoscopist. It provides interrupted suction for evacuation of fluid or blood that can be used for laboratory evaluation (Figs. 7.1 and 7.2).

*Manufacturer: Karl Storz, Endoscopy-America, Inc.

The technique of emergency laparoscopy is in most respects similar to routine diagnostic laparoscopy (for further details, see Chapter 1).

LAPAROSCOPIC FINDINGS

Hemoperitoneum

It is important to observe the presence or absence of blood within the peritoneal cavity. The location and quantity of blood are important.

The distribution of blood within the abdomen can provide clues to the location or the bleeding site. In the case of pelvic fractures, this will be confined to the pelvic area. Pelvic fracture is the most common cause of false-positive lavage results.

Quantitative assessment in the abdominal cavity is difficult, but an impression can be gained with some experience. We decided to divide hemoperitoneum into minimal, moderate, and severe categories.

The refinement and accuracy of the observations made by emergency laparoscopy provide far greater latitude in the decision-making process in hemoperitoneum. This is a distinct advantage, in comparison with peritoneal lavage alone.

Minimal Hemoperitoneum

A small amount of blood will be discovered in the lateral peritoneal gutter, or streaks of blood will be seen between intestinal loops. If there is no increase in the small volume of blood during the procedure and if the search for bleeding site has been unrevealing, then the patient can usually be treated conservatively and observed likewise. If a bleeding site is found, the bleeding may amount to a minimal ooze or may be stopped completely. In our experience, a bleeding site is found only in 50% of patients classified as having a minimal hemoperitoneum. Extremely small volumes of blood in the peritoneal cavity, as in this case, are nevertheless sufficient to produce a positive lavage.

Moderate Hemoperitoneum

If 10 to 20 ml of blood can be found in one of the lateral gutters, the patient is considered to have a moderate hemoperitoneum. In such cases, the second trocar should be introduced immediately. The suction coagulation palpation probe should be introduced, and the hemoperitoneum evacuated. A thorough and systematic search is initiated, making use of a suction cannula as a palpation manipulation probe. If organ injury with bleeding is discovered (e.g., liver laceration), the site of injury should be observed carefully. If the bleeding is brisk, surgical intervention is indicated. If the bleeding site is not found after 5 or 10 minutes of diligent search and the gutter is refilled with blood to the previous level, the bleeding vessel is probably not within the range of laparoscopy; surgical intervention should be considered. If a small laceration is oozing, and a small amount of blood is found or evidence of cessation of bleeding is observed or blood clots are seen in the vicinity of laceration but there is no active bleeding, then patients can be managed by observation alone. This suction coagulation palpation probe may be used to aspirate blood from an oozing lesion to access the rate of blood loss. In selected cases, coagulation may also be applied. If injuries are found that require immediate operation, precise location of the injury facilitates the selection of the optimal incision.

Severe Hemoperitoneum

If aspiration with a pneumoperitoneum needle clearly results in blood in the syringe on two or three attempts, or if this does not result in aspiration of blood but laparoscopic observation displays intestinal loops floating in or surrounded by a pool of blood, then the indication for immediate operation is obvious. Blood in the lateral gutters to a depth of two or more finger breadths should also be classified as a severe hemoperitoneum.

ORGAN PERFORATIONS

In cases of perforation of one of the hollow intraabdominal organs, a yellowish fluid will be seen in the gutters. This can be aspirated and sent for laboratory analysis. However, these findings in general are consistent with perforation and represent an indication for exploration.

If several hours have lapsed between the trauma and the examination, the actual injury may not be seen. However, it may be suspected because of indirect findings such as a conglomerate or omentum in one particular area or small aggregation of edematous hyperemic intestinal loops. A palpation probe can be of help by moving such loops or omentum.

Perforation with the retroperitoneal segment of the duodenum or pancreatic injuries will escape detection at laparoscopy. Fortunately, these lesions are rare, and other diagnostic measures will have to clarify this clinical picture.

SPLENIC INJURIES

Splenic injuries are characterized by accumulation of blood in the left gutter. A normal-sized spleen is seldom seen in the left upper quadrant because it is usually covered by the omentum. The omentum covering the spleen is elevated by a pool of blood or blood clots. Splenic injuries can have serious consequences and often are an indication for splenectomy. However, conservation of the spleen is also desirable and can be accomplished in selected cases.[6] In some cases of splenic trauma, the laparoscopic appearance is a minimal hemoperitoneum in the area but without a significant bulge or bluish color of the omentum lying over the spleen. This assessment requires judgment and experience. However, if the injury is found to be minimal at laparoscopy and the patient's vital signs are stable, conservative management with very careful observation can be initiated even if the spleen scan can denote splenic injury.

LIVER INJURY

Deceleration injuries are frequently characterized by laceration on the anterior surface or dome of the liver lobe and in the vicinity of the round or falciform ligament. These areas are easily observed at laparoscopy. The undersurface of the liver can also be inspected with the aid of a palpation probe by gently lifting up segments of the right lobe and the entire left lobe. If a laceration is found, the telescope is advanced, and the area is observed closely for a few minutes. In the case of small oozing laceration, compression or coagulation may be employed. However, if at the end of observation, bleeding persists, laparotomy should be considered.

PENETRATING INJURY

Laparoscopy is not performed for gunshot wounds of the abdomen. However, a wound produced by stab incisions in which it is uncertain as to whether the peritoneal cavity was entered is not a contraindication to laparoscopy. A laparoscopy may be of assistance in determining the presence or extent of intraabdominal injury as a result of a stab wound. Our approach is as follows: the skin is temporarily closed to provide a seal for the pneumoperitoneum. Laparoscopic observation in the region of the presumed penetration is highly accurate with respect to excluding or confirming that the parietal peritoneum has been penetrated. If inspection of the parietal surface indicates that the abdomen was entered, the area underlying the penetration site should be inspected with the aid of a palpation probe. Loops of bowel should be lifted and pushed gently aside to look for signs of bleeding, serosal injuries, leakage of fluid, and other signs of perforation or hemorrhage.

RESULTS

We performed emergency laparoscopy consecutively in 129 blunt abdominal traumas, and the results are summarized below.

Negative Laparoscopy (No Operation)

There were 72 cases (55.8%) in this category. No hemoperitoneum or other abnormalities were discovered, and none of these patients subsequently required exploratory laparotomy.

Positive Laparoscopy (No Operation)

Minimal or moderate hemoperitoneum was found in 33 cases (25.5%). However, there was no identified injury, but only minimal lacerations were seen on these patients. The patients were, therefore, observed in the Intensive Care Unit. Only one patient required laparotomy subsequent to this decision. In this case, a sealed perforation of the sigmoid colon near the rectus sigmoid junction was overlooked.

Positive Laparoscopy (Operation)

Severe hemoperitoneum was present at emergency laparoscopy in 24 patients (18.6%), all of whom underwent surgery. The source of bleeding or perforation was found endoscopically and confirmed at surgery in all but one patient. The 24 cases included 3 liver lacerations, 11 splenic injuries (in 6 patients, the spleen was saved by splenorrhaphia), 4 organ perforations, and 6 carrier bleeders.

COMPLICATIONS

In one patient, a minimum amount of hemoperitoneum was interpreted as being caused by injuries or omentum during trocar insertion. Fresh coagulum was seen in the area. Observation only was required.

DISCUSSION

Emergency laparoscopy is extremely helpful in avoiding unnecessary abdominal explorations in cases of hemoperitoneum in which peritoneal lavage reveals intraabdominal bleeding. Most of our patients who sustained multiple injuries and were at high surgical risk were elderly patients. Abdominal surgery in these patients would have increased postoperative morbidity and, therefore, it was important to avoid any unnecessary operations. The technique of emergency laparoscopy is not difficult. It provides a safe, fast, and accurate method of diagnosis in cases in which the presence and/or extent of intraabdominal injuries are uncertain or unknown. In our experience, the use of emergency laparoscopy has avoided surgery in a significant number of patients. Unfortunately, traumatic injury is a common occurrence that results in significant loss of life and morbidity. A complete and accurate evaluation is of great importance in such cases, and in this respect, emergency laparoscopy can play a significant role.

REFERENCES

1. Root HD, Hauser CW, McKinley CR, et al.: Diagnostic peritoneal lavage. *Surgery* 57: 633–637, 1965.
2. Sherwood R, Berci G, Austin E, et al.: Minilaparoscopy for blunt abdominal trauma. *Arch Surg* 115: 672–674, 1980.
3. Federle MP, Brooke J, Crass A, et al.: Computed tomography in blunt abdominal trauma. *Arch Surg* 117: 645–650, 1982.
4. Gazzaniga AB, Stanton WW, Bartlett G: Laparoscopy in the diagnosis of blunt and penetrating injuries to the abdomen. *Am J Surg* 131: 315–318, 1976.
5. Berci G, Dunkelman D, Michel S, et al.: Emergency laparoscopy. *Am J Surg* 146: 261–265, 1983.
6. Morgenstern L, Shapiro S.: Techniques of splenic conservation. *Arch Surg* 114: 449–454, 1979.

Appendix

SUGGESTED READING

1. Berci G, Cushieri A: Practical Laparoscopy. London, Bailliere Tindall, 1986.
2. Boyce HW Jr, Palmer E: Techniques of Clinical Gastroenterology. Springfield, Charles C. Thomas, 1975.
3. Dagnini G: Clinical Laparoscopy. Padua, Piccin, 1980.
4. Dubois R, Icard P, Berthelot G, et al: Coelioscopic Cholecystectomy. *Ann Surg* 211: 60–62, 1990.
5. Ishida H, Furukawa Y, Kuroda H, et al: Laparoscopic Observation and Biopsy of the Pancreas. *Endoscopy* 13(2): 69–73, 1981.
6. Lightdale CJ: Clinical Applications of Laparoscopy in Patients with Malignant Neoplasms. *Gastro Endosc* 28(2): 99–102, 1982.
7. Salky BA, Bauer JJ, Gelernt IM, et al: The Use of Laparoscopy in Retroperitoneal Pathology. *Gastro Endosc* 34: 227–230, 1988.

INDEX

A

Abdominal cavity, normal, 12
Abdominal mass, 45–58
  accuracy of laparoscopy in, 45–46
Abdominal pain, hepatic metastasis and, 78
Abscess
  amebic, therapeutic laparoscopy in, 114
  pericholecystic, 26–27
Acquired immune deficiency syndrome (AIDS), 20–21
Adenocarcinoma
  adrenal, hepatic metastasis and, 97
  colloid, 48
  colonic, 47
  hepatic, 74, 77–81, 86, 89, 92, 97
  mucin-producing, 81
  pancreatic, 57–58
    hepatic metastasis and, 90, 96
  with psammoma bodies, ascites and, 107
  rectal, ascites and, 110
  signet-ring, ascites and, 111
Adenoma, hepatic, 61
Adhesion
  lysis of, 40–41
  single-band, 39–40
  therapeutic laparoscopy in, 123, 126–129
Amebic abscess, therapeutic laparoscopy in, 114
Anesthesia, 113
  administration of, 8
Anorexia, 97
Appendicitis, 18–25
  differential diagnosis of, 32–36
Appendix, therapeutic laparoscopy in disorders of, 123–125
Ascites, 10, 99–11
  benign, 100–103
  bloody, 106
  exudative, 99–100, 102, 110
  malignant, 103–111
  tense, 100–102, 103
  transudative, 99

B

Biliary colic, therapeutic laparoscopy in, 137–143
Biliary tract adenocarcinoma, hepatic metastasis and, 78–80
Blood clot, therapeutic laparoscopy in, 129–130
Body weight, as factor in laparoscopy, 9
Breast cancer
  ascites and, 108–109
  hepatic metastasis and, 76, 88

C

Carbon dioxide, 8
Carcinoma, *see also* Adenocarcinoma
  gallbladder, hepatic metastasis and, 93–94
  hepatic, 73–76, 88, 90
  hepatocellular, ascites and, 106
  ovarian
    ascites and, 103
    hepatic metastasis and, 92
  signet-ring, ascites and, 104
  transitional cell, 56
  undifferentiated, ascites and, 110–111
Cecal enteritis, 20–22
Cholecystectomy, laparoscopic, 137–143
Cholecystitis, 26–28
  chronic, 38
Cirrhosis, 70–71, 82
  ascites and, 100–101
Coagulapathy, as contraindication in laparoscopy, 2
Colic, biliary, therapeutic laparoscopy in, 137–143
Colloid adenocarcinoma, 48
Colon, 15, 16
Colon cancer, 47
  hepatic metastasis and, 77–78, 85–86, 88
Corpus luteal cyst, 21
Crohn's disease, 36
Cyst
corpus luteal, 21
  ecchinococcal, 73
  hepatic, 16
    benign, 64, 69–70
  splenic, therapeutic laparoscopy in, 118
Cytological examination, in ascites, 99

D

Diabetes, 96
  ascites and, 101
Dialysis catheter, placement of, 131
Diverticulitis, transverse colon, 30–32

E

Ecchinococcal cyst, 73
Endometriosis, 38
Enteritis
  acute, 24
  cecal, 20–22
Eosinophilic gastritis, 95

F

Falciform ligament, 11
Fallopian tube, hydrosalpinx of, 37
Fiberoptic cable, 3
Fibrotic appendix, therapeutic laparoscopy in, 123
Fitzhugh-Curtis syndrome, 36–37
Forceps, 3

G

Gallbladder, 16
Gallbladder carcinoma, hepatic metastasis and, 79–80, 93–94
Ganglioneuroma, 49
Gastritis, eosinophilic, 95
Gastrointestinal disease, hepatic metastasis and, 81

H

Hemangioma, hepatic, 60, 63, 66–68
Hematoma, hepatic, with splenomegaly, 84
Hemoperitoneum, 25–26, 148–149
  pelvic, 19
Hemorrhage, spontaneous, with hepatic hepatoma, 81
Hepatic adenoma, 61
Hepatic carcinoma, 74
Hepatic cyst, benign, 64, 69–70
Hepatic hemangioma, 60, 63, 66–68
Hepatic necrosis, 61–62
Hepatic sarcoid, 65
Hepatic schistosomiasis, 68
Hepatocellular carcinoma, ascites and, 106
Hepatoma, hepatic, 82, 95
  with hemorrhage, 81
Hernia, 1
Histiocytic lymphoma, 53

Hodgkin's lymphoma, hepatic metastasis and, 87
Hook-scissor, 3
Hydrosalpinx, of fallopian tube, 37
Hyperplasia
  appendiceal inflammation and, 125
  nodular, focal, 66–67

I
Illumination, 3
Infarction, omentum, 29, 31
Infection, as contraindication for laparoscopy, 2
Injection, sites for, 7–8
Instrumentation, in laparoscopy, 2–6
Insufflation
  gas for, 8–9
  technique in, 9–10
Intestine, small, 14, 15
Intraabdominal examination, emergency laparoscopy in, 145–152

K
Krukenberg's tumor, 47

L
Laparoscopy
  accuracy of, 45–46, 60, 100
  contraindications for, 1–2
  indications for, 1
  instruments for, 147
  technique in, 6–16
  therapeutic, 113–152
    emergency, 145–152
Leiomyoma, 47
Leiomyosarcoma, hepatic metastasis and, 82
Leukemia, hepatic metastasis and, 83
Lidocaine, 8
Ligament, falciform, 11
Liver disease, 59–98; *see also* Hepatic *specific diseases*
  accuracy of laparoscopy in, 59–60
  benign, 60–72
  indications for laparoscopy in, 59
  malignant, 73–98
Liver injury, laparoscopy in, 150
Lymphoma, 51
  histiocytic, 53
  Hodgkin's, hepatic metastatis and, 87
  non-Hodgkin's, 45–46, 51–56

M
Malignant disease, 45; *see also specific malignancies*
  ascites and, 103–111
  benign disease versus, 28
  hepatic, 73–98
Melanoma, hepatic metastasis and, 84–85
Mesothelioma, 105–106
  peritoneal, ascites and, 104
Minilaparotomy, 60
Mucocele, of appendix, 35–36
Myeloid metaplasia, splenomegaly and, 84

N
Necrosis, hepatic, 61–62
Nitrous oxide, 8
Non-Hodgkin's lymphoma, 45–46, 51–56

O
Obese patient, Veress insufflation needle for, 2
Omentum infarction, 29, 31
Ovarian carcinoma
  ascites and, 103
  hepatic metastasis and, 92

P
Pain, abdominal, 17–43
  accuracy of laparoscopy in, 17–18
  acute, 18–25
  chronic, 17–18, 28–43
  right upper quadrant, 25–28
Palpating probe, 3
Pancreas, adenocarcinoma of, 57–58
  hepatic metastasis and, 90
Paracentesis, in ascites, 104, 106, 110–111
Pelvic hemoperitoneum, 19
Pelvic kidney, 42
Pelvic view, 12
Perforation, organ, laparoscopy in, 149
Pericholecystic abscess, 26–27
Peritoneal mesothelioma, ascites and, 104
Photographic documentation, in laparoscopy, 3, 6
Pneumotosis intestinalis, segmental, 42–43
Pressure, intraabdominal, 9–10, 11
Psammoma bodies, ovarian carcinoma and, 92
Puncture site, in laparoscopy, 7–8

R
Rectal adenocarcinoma, ascites and, 110
Retroperitoneal mass, 45

S
Sarcoid, hepatic, 65
Sarcoma, spindle cell, 46–47
Schistosomiasis, 68
  hepatic, 68
Sigmoid colon, 15
Signet-ring adenocarcinoma, ascites and, 111
Spindle cell sarcoma, 46–47
Splenic cyst, therapeutic laparoscopy in, 118
Splenic injury, laparoscopy in, 149–150
Splenomegaly, with myeloid metaplasis, 84
Stab wound, laparoscopy in, 150
Surgery
  laparoscopic, 113–152
    emergency, 145–152
  previous
    as contraindication for laparoscopy, 2
    puncture site in patient with, 8

T
Table, for laparoscopy, 6–7
Telescope, size of, 2, 3
Tenckhoff dialysis catheter, placement of, 131
Tenia coli, 14
Transitional cell carcinoma, metastatic, 56
Transverse colon diverticulitis, 30–32
Trocar, 3, 10, 11
Tuberculosis peritonitis, ascites and, 102

U
Umbilical approach, 8
Urinary bladder, 15
Uterus, 15

V
Veress needle, 2–3, 8–11
  sites for insertion of, 7–8

W
Wheal, anesthetic, 12

Y
Yersinia, 21–22